Accelerating the Use of Findings from Patient-Centered Outcomes Research in Clinical Practice to Improve Health and Health Care

Crystal Bell, Lyle Carrera, Austen Applegate, and Joe Alper, *Rapporteurs*

Board on Health Care Services

Health and Medicine Division

Proceedings of a Workshop Series

THE NATIONAL ACADEMIES PRESS 500 Fifth Street, NW Washington, DC 20001

This activity was supported by contracts between the National Academy of Sciences and the Department of Health and Human Services Agency for Healthcare Research and Quality. Any opinions, findings, conclusions, or recommendations expressed in this publication do not necessarily reflect the views of any organization or agency that provided support for the project.

International Standard Book Number-13: 978-0-309-69513-8
International Standard Book Number-10: 0-309-69513-9
Digital Object Identifier: https://doi.org/10.17226/26753

This publication is available from the National Academies Press, 500 Fifth Street, NW, Keck 360, Washington, DC 20001; (800) 624-6242 or (202) 334-3313; http://www.nap.edu.

Copyright 2022 by the National Academy of Sciences. National Academies of Sciences, Engineering, and Medicine and National Academies Press and the graphical logos for each are all trademarks of the National Academy of Sciences. All rights reserved.

Printed in the United States of America.

Suggested citation: National Academies of Sciences, Engineering, and Medicine. 2022. *Accelerating the use of findings from patient-centered outcomes research in clinical practice to improve health and health care: Proceedings of a workshop series.* Washington, DC: The National Academies Press. https://doi.org/10.17226/26753.

The **National Academy of Sciences** was established in 1863 by an Act of Congress, signed by President Lincoln, as a private, nongovernmental institution to advise the nation on issues related to science and technology. Members are elected by their peers for outstanding contributions to research. Dr. Marcia McNutt is president.

The **National Academy of Engineering** was established in 1964 under the charter of the National Academy of Sciences to bring the practices of engineering to advising the nation. Members are elected by their peers for extraordinary contributions to engineering. Dr. John L. Anderson is president.

The **National Academy of Medicine** (formerly the Institute of Medicine) was established in 1970 under the charter of the National Academy of Sciences to advise the nation on medical and health issues. Members are elected by their peers for distinguished contributions to medicine and health. Dr. Victor J. Dzau is president.

The three Academies work together as the **National Academies of Sciences, Engineering, and Medicine** to provide independent, objective analysis and advice to the nation and conduct other activities to solve complex problems and inform public policy decisions. The National Academies also encourage education and research, recognize outstanding contributions to knowledge, and increase public understanding in matters of science, engineering, and medicine.

Learn more about the National Academies of Sciences, Engineering, and Medicine at **www.nationalacademies.org**.

Consensus Study Reports published by the National Academies of Sciences, Engineering, and Medicine document the evidence-based consensus on the study's statement of task by an authoring committee of experts. Reports typically include findings, conclusions, and recommendations based on information gathered by the committee and the committee's deliberations. Each report has been subjected to a rigorous and independent peer-review process and it represents the position of the National Academies on the statement of task.

Proceedings published by the National Academies of Sciences, Engineering, and Medicine chronicle the presentations and discussions at a workshop, symposium, or other event convened by the National Academies. The statements and opinions contained in proceedings are those of the participants and are not endorsed by other participants, the planning committee, or the National Academies.

Rapid Expert Consultations published by the National Academies of Sciences, Engineering, and Medicine are authored by subject-matter experts on narrowly focused topics that can be supported by a body of evidence. The discussions contained in rapid expert consultations are considered those of the authors and do not contain policy recommendations. Rapid expert consultations are reviewed by the institution before release.

For information about other products and activities of the National Academies, please visit www.nationalacademies.org/about/whatwedo.

PLANNING COMMITTEE FOR A WORKSHOP ON ACCELERATING THE USE OF FINDINGS FROM PATIENT-CENTERED OUTCOMES RESEARCH IN CLINICAL PRACTICE TO IMPROVE HEALTH AND HEALTH CARE[1]

LAUREN S. HUGHES (*Chair*), Associate Professor of Family Medicine and State Policy Director of the Farley Health Policy Center, University of Colorado

JEN F. BROWN, Co-Founder and Co-Director, Alliance for Research in Chicagoland Communities, Northwestern University

MEGAN D. DOUGLAS, Assistant Professor, Department of Community Health and Preventive Medicine and Director of Research and Policy, National Center for Primary Care, Morehouse School of Medicine

CATHERINE L. KOTHARI, Associate Professor and Population Health Scientist, Division of Epidemiology and Biostatistics, Homer Stryker MD School of Medicine, Western Michigan University

MEGHAN B. LANE-FALL, Vice Chair of Inclusion, Diversity, and Equity; David E. Longnecker Associate Professor of Anesthesiology and Critical Care; and Associate Professor, Biostatistics, Epidemiology, and Informatics, University of Pennsylvania Perelman School of Medicine; Founding Co-Director, Penn Center for Perioperative Outcomes Research and Transformation; Vice President, Anesthesia Patient Safety Foundation

CARA E. NIKOLAJSKI, Director of Research Design and Implementation, UPMC Center for High-Value Health Care, University of Pittsburgh Medical Center

BRIAN RIVERS, Professor and Director, Cancer Health Equity Institute, Morehouse School of Medicine

SARAH H. SCHOLLE, Vice President, Research and Analysis, National Committee for Quality Assurance

---

[1] The National Academies of Sciences, Engineering, and Medicine's planning committees are solely responsible for organizing the workshop, identifying topics, and choosing speakers. The responsibility for the published Proceedings of a Workshop Series rests with the workshop rapporteurs and the institution.

Project Staff

CRYSTAL BELL, Associate Program Officer
AUSTEN APPLEGATE, Research Associate (since May 2022)
LORI BRENIG, Research Associate (May 2022–July 2022)
TORRIE BROWN, Senior Program Assistant (May 2022–July 2022)
LYLE CARRERA, Research Associate (since June 2022)
JOSEPH GOODMAN, Senior Program Assistant (May 2022–July 2022)
RUKSHANA GUPTA, Senior Program Assistant (March 2022–June 2022)
SIHAM IDRIS, Program Assistant (December 2022–March 2022)
SHARYL NASS, Senior Board Director
ARZOO TAYYEB, Finance Business Partner

Consultant

JOE ALPER, Consulting Writer

Reviewers

This Proceedings of a Workshop Series was reviewed in draft form by individuals chosen for their diverse perspectives and technical expertise. The purpose of this independent review is to provide candid and critical comments that will assist the National Academies of Sciences, Engineering, and Medicine in making each published proceedings as sound as possible and to ensure that it meets the institutional standards for quality, objectivity, evidence, and responsiveness to the charge. The review comments and draft manuscript remain confidential to protect the integrity of the process.

We thank the following individuals for their review of this proceedings:

WALETHA WASSON, University of Tennessee
MARGARET I. GRADIE, University of Massachusetts Amherst
JEFFERY ULLMAN, Stanford University (Emeritus)

Although the reviewers listed above provided many constructive comments and suggestions, they were not asked to endorse the content of the proceedings nor did they see the final draft before its release. The review of this proceedings was overseen by **KATHRYN McDONALD,** Johns Hopkins University. She was responsible for making certain that an independent examination of this proceedings was carried out in accordance with standards of the National Academies and that all review comments were carefully considered. Responsibility for the final content rests entirely with the rapporteurs and the National Academies.

Acknowledgments

The National Academies of Sciences, Engineering, and Medicine's Board on Health Care Services thanks planning committee chair Lauren S. Hughes for her valuable contributions to the development and organization of this workshop. The board wishes to thank all the members of the planning committee, who collaborated to ensure a workshop complete with informative presentations and rich discussions. Finally, the board thanks the speakers and moderators, who generously shared their expertise and their time with workshop participants.

Contents

BOX, FIGURES, AND TABLE   xv

ACRONYMS AND ABBREVIATIONS   xvii

1 INTRODUCTION   1

2 WORKSHOP 1 KEYNOTE: COMMUNITY HEALTH WORKERS   3
Introduction to Workshop, 3
Sponsor Remarks from AHRQ, 4
Community Health Workers: A Link Between Provider and Patient, 5
Discussion, 10

3 WORKSHOP 1, SESSION 1: DEVELOPING A COORDINATED INTERDISCIPLINARY APPROACH TO DECISION MAKING AROUND WHERE TO FOCUS AHRQ'S PCORTF INVESTMENTS   11
A Focus on Goals and Authentic Partnerships, 12
Practice-Based Research Networks and Community Engagement, 14
Discussion, 16

4   **WORKSHOP 1, SESSION 2: TRAINING PCOR
    INVESTIGATORS**   19
    Collaborations for Training Community-Based Researchers, 19
    Educational Training for the Next Generation of Investigators, 22
    Discussion, 25

5   **WORKSHOP 1, SESSION 3: SUSTAINABLE STRATEGIES
    AND DIGITAL TOOLS TO EXPAND
    IMPLEMENTATION OF PCOR FINDINGS**   29
    Using the Learning Collaborative Approach for Implementing
      and Scaling Innovation, 29
    Person-Centered and Sustainable Digital Reproductive Health
      Interventions, 32
    Engaging People in Innovative Digital Interventions, 34
    Discussion, 37
    Closing Summary of Workshop 1, 39

6   **WORKSHOP 2 KEYNOTE: COMMUNITY
    ENGAGEMENT IN PCOR FOR HEALTH EQUITY**   41
    Introduction, 41
    Meaningful Community Engagement to Advance Health
      Equity in Health Systems Transformation, 42
    Discussion, 44

7   **WORKSHOP 2, SESSION 1: POSSIBILITIES FOR AHRQ–
    ASPE–PCORI COLLABORATIONS TO IMPROVE
    HEALTH EQUITY**   47
    The Role of Data in Health Equity, 48
    Strengthening the Primary Care System While Advancing
      Health Equity, 48
    Addressing Health Equity Through Dissemination and
      Implementation Science, 51
    Community Partnerships in Research, 54
    Discussion, 56

8   **WORKSHOP 2, SESSION 2: OPPORTUNITIES FOR
    AHRQ, ASPE, PCORI COLLABORATIONS TO
    IMPROVE SUSTAINABILITY OF THEIR EFFORTS**   59
    Maintaining Partnerships for Sustainable Data Collection, 59

CONTENTS *xiii*

    State-Level Data Collaborations, 61
    AHRQ–ASPE–PCORI Collaborations to Improve Effort
        Sustainability, 64
    Discussion, 66
    Closing Summary of Workshop 2, 69

9 WORKSHOP 3, SESSION 1: MEASURING THE
    IMPACT OF DISSEMINATION PROJECTS   71
    Workshop Introduction, 71
    Evaluating Dissemination and Implementation Projects, 72
    Using Digital Tools for Dissemination and Implelentation in
        the Community, 73
    Community Engagement in Evaluating the Effectiveness of
        Dissemination and Implementation Projects, 74
    Discussion, 77

10 WORKSHOP 3, SESSION 2: MEASURING THE
     IMPACT OF DISSEMINATION PROJECTS PART 2   81
     Generalizability and Temporality in Assessing Effect, 81
     Clinician Engagement With a Breast Reconstruction
         Decision Support Tool, 84
     Incorporating PCOR into Clinical Practice:
         A Digital Technology Case Study, 87
     Discussion, 90
     Closing Summary of Workshop 3, 93

11 WORKSHOP 4, SESSION 1: EFFECTIVE
     COMMUNICATION TOOLS   95
     Workshop Introduction, 96
     Translating Policy and Patient-Centered Outcomes Outside
         the Institutional Bubble, 96
     Perspectives in Health Communication, 97
     How Law and Policy Can Advance Health Equity, 100
     Discussion, 102

12 WORKSHOP 4, SESSION 2: INFORMING EVIDENCE-
     BASED POLICY MAKING   107
     Conceptualizing and Conducting Policy-Relevant Research, 108

Changing Access to Care for Undocumented Immigrants
with Data, 110
Dissemination Research to Promote Evidence-Informed Policy
Making, 114
Discussion, 118
Closing Summary of Workshop 4, 120

REFERENCES 123

APPENDIXES
A STATEMENT OF TASK 133
B WORKSHOP AGENDAS 135
C BIOGRAPHICAL SKETCHES OF THE SPEAKERS 141
D AHRQ'S PCORTF INVESTMENT STRATEGIC
   FRAMEWORK 155

Box, Figures, and Table

BOX

7-1 One Community's Guiding Principles for University Engagement, 55

FIGURES

2-1 Community health workers address all stages of health inequity, 6
2-2 Project IMPaCT's ordered process that allows community health workers to achieve success consistently, 9

5-1 Conceptual model for experimental therapeutics to target engagement as a mediating mechanism for digital mental health, 35
5-2 Implementation strategies for digital mental health, 36

6-1 A conceptual model for assessing community engagement, 43

9-1 Total referrals (left) and referrals per 1,000 cases (right) for use of mAbs in Colorado as of July 31, 2021, 76

10-1 A large difference in the slope of the enrollment versus risk relationship indicates that the incentive results in undue inducement (graph is for illustrative purposes and does not represent data from an actual study), 83

10-2 A large difference in the slope of the enrollment versus incentive size according to economic status indicates that the incentive results in unjust inducement (graph is for illustrative purposes and does not represent data from an actual study), 83

10-3 Evolving applications of digital technology in health and health care, 88

11-1 The public health impact pyramid, 98

11-2 The role of law in advancing AHRQ's crosscutting strategies, 101

12-1 Medicaid-covered provision of standard dialysis for undocumented immigrants in 2019, 112

TABLE

12-1 Audience Segmentation According to Beliefs About Mental Health and Substance Use Disorder, 117

Acronyms and Abbreviations

AHRQ   Agency for Healthcare Research and Quality
AI/ML   artificial intelligence and machine learning
ASPE   Assistant Secretary for Planning and Evaluation

BETTER   Behavioral Economics to Transform Trial Enrollment Representativeness

CBO   community-based organization
CCTSI   Clinical and Translational Sciences Institute
CDC   Centers for Disease Control and Prevention
CDU   Charles R. Drew University of Medicine and Science
CHECS   Collaborations for Health and Empowered Community-Based Scientists
CMS   Centers for Medicare and Medicaid Services
COM-B   Capability, Opportunity, and Motivation Model of Behavior
CU   University of Colorado

EnCoRE   Enhancing Community Health Center Patient-Centered Outcomes Research Engagement
EHR   electronic health record
FDA   Food and Drug Administration

HHS   Department of Health and Human Services
HRSA   Health Resources and Services Administration

ICU	intensive care unit
IMPaCT	Individualized Management for Patient-Centered Targets
mAb	Monoclonal Antibodies
MODRN	Medicaid Outcomes Distributed Research Network
NAM	National Academy of Medicine
NAMCS	National Ambulatory Medical Care Survey
NCPC	National Center for Primary Care
NIH	National Institutes of Health
OMB	Office of Management and Budget
PBRN	practice-based research network
PCOR	patient-centered outcomes research
PCORI	Patient-Centered Outcomes Research Institute
PCORTF	Patient-Centered Outcomes Research Trust Fund
PDSA	Plan-Do-Study-Act
RE-AIM	Reach, Effectiveness, Adoption, Implementation, and Maintenance
RETAIN	Randomized Evaluation of Trial Acceptance by Incentive
SHADAC	State Health Access Data Assistance Center
SNOCAP	State Networks of Colorado Ambulatory Practices & Partners
T-MSIS	Transformed Medicaid Statistical Information System
UPMC	University of Pittsburgh Medical Center
UC	University of California
VHA	Veterans Health Administration

1

Introduction[1]

In 2010, as part of the Patient Protection and Affordable Care Act, Congress established the Patient-Centered Outcomes Research Trust Fund (PCORTF). PCORTF funds are divided between three entities charged with meeting the goals of the PCORTF, Patient Centered Outcomes Research Institute (PCORI), Agency for Healthcare Research and Quality (AHRQ), and the Department of Health and Human Services' (DHHS) Office of the Assistant Secretary for Planning and Evaluation (ASPE). Congress's goal was to improve the quality and relevance of evidence available to help patients and their caregivers, clinicians, payers, and policy makers make better-informed health care decisions by expanding and improving comparative effectiveness research through patient-centered outcomes research (PCOR).[2] PCOR studies consider the questions and outcomes that are meaningful to patients to compare the effectiveness of different prevention, diagnostic, and treatment options. PCOR also increases a patient's involvement in their care by provid-

---

[1] The planning committee's role was limited to planning the workshop, and the Proceedings of a Workshop Series has been prepared by the workshop rapporteurs as a factual summary of what occurred at the workshop. Statements, recommendations, and opinions expressed are those of individual presenters and participants and are not necessarily endorsed or verified by the National Academies of Sciences, Engineering, and Medicine, and they should not be construed as reflecting any group consensus.

[2] Patient-Centered Outcomes Research (PCOR) compares the impact of two or more preventive, diagnostic, treatment, or health care delivery approaches on health outcomes, including those that are meaningful to patients (AHRQ, 2016).

ing them an opportunity to evaluate the quality, outcomes, and effectiveness of health care treatments and intervention, especially in areas where there is poor existing clinical evidence.

AHRQ tasked the National Academies of Sciences, Engineering, and Medicine's Board on Health Care Services to host a series of public workshops that explore ways of accelerating the use of PCOR findings in clinical practice to improve health and health care. The resulting virtual workshop series, Accelerating the Use of Findings from Patient-Centered Outcomes Research in Clinical Practice to Improve Health and Health Care: A Workshop Series, comprised four virtual workshops that took place on June 9, June 17, July 1, and July 6 of 2022. The workshops' presentations and discussions examined topics in four main categories that were described in the project's statement of task:

1. Ways to revise and improve AHRQ's proposed strategic plan, priorities, and strategies to make them clearer and more likely to lead to funding high-impact and complementary projects while being consistent with the congressional mandate for investing funds from PCORTF.
2. Ways to measure progress and the effect of AHRQ's PCORTF investments as a whole on meeting its goals in the near, short, and long term.
3. Ways to better align priorities and strategies and to create complementary collaborations between the agencies charged with using PCORTF to improve patient-centered outcomes research and practice so as to increase the impact of AHRQ's PCORTF investments and their potential to sustainably reduce disparities.
4. Ways AHRQ can apply communication science to improve dissemination of evidence, gaps in evidence, and policy gaps to inform health policies and decision makers at local, state, and federal levels.

This Proceedings of a Workshop Series summarizes the presentations and discussions. The speakers, panelists, and workshop participants presented a broad range of views and ideas. Appendix A contains the workshop statement of task. Appendix B contains the workshop agendas, Appendix C contains biographical sketches for members of the planning committee and the speakers for all four workshops, and Appendix D contains AHRQ's proposed strategic framework for its PCORTF investments. The workshop speakers' presentations (as PDF and audio files) have been archived online.[3]

---

[3] All workshop speaker presentations are available here: https://www.nationalacademies.org/our-work/accelerating-the-use-of-findings-from-patient-centered-outcomes-research-in-clinical-practice-to-improve-health-and-health-care-a-workshop-series#sectionPastEvents (accessed September 28, 2022).

2

Workshop 1 Keynote: Community Health Workers

Key Messages Presented by Individual Speakers

- Community health workers are the link who can help health care providers see and understand the whole picture of their patients' lives, not just the part they see in their offices. (Burke)
- An ordered process of hiring, training, working, supervising, and evaluating provides community health workers with the tools and knowledge to achieve consistent, positive results. (Kangovi)
- Sustainable and adequate funding for community health worker programs rather than the current patchwork of grants and demonstration projects is needed for the nation to realize the full value that community health workers can create. (Kangovi)

INTRODUCTION TO WORKSHOP

Lauren Hughes, associate professor of family medicine and state policy director of the Farley Health Policy Center at the University of Colorado, explained that the first workshop will explore the Agency for Healthcare Research and Quality's (AHRQ's) proposed priorities and strategies to make them clearer and more likely to lead to high-impact funding and projects, while also being consistent with the congressional mandate to invest funds from the Patient-Centered Outcomes Research Trust Fund (PCORTF). The day's sessions began with a keynote address on the important role community health workers can play in equitable implementation of patient-centered outcomes research (PCOR). The sessions then discussed innovative models of care delivery, approaches to guiding decision-making regarding PCORTF investments, how to train PCOR investigators, and the use of digital tools to expand implementation of PCOR findings.

SPONSOR REMARKS FROM AHRQ

Following Hughes's introductory remarks, Karin Rhodes, AHRQ's chief implementation officer, provided additional background on PCORTF and AHRQ's role. Rhodes provided some definitions before discussing PCORTF's mandate. PCOR, she explained, provides decision makers with objective scientific evidence on comparative effectiveness of different treatments, services, and other interventions used in health care, while PCORTF, which receives most of its funds from a tax on private insurance plans, provides funding to support dissemination, training, and data infrastructure for PCOR. She explained that Congress mandated that 80 percent of trust fund spending would go to the Patient-Centered Outcomes Research Institute (PCORI) to conduct comparative effectiveness research. AHRQ receives 16 percent of trust fund spending to disseminate this evidence into practice as well as train health services researchers, and the Assistant Secretary for Planning and Evaluation (ASPE) at the U.S. Department of Health and Human Services receives the remaining 4 percent to develop the data infrastructure for PCOR.

She explained that Congress reauthorized PCORTF in 2020, and PCORI, AHRQ, and ASPE are all now engaged in strategic planning for the next 10 years. Rhodes noted that unlike most congressionally authorized funds, which have to be spent in the year Congress authorizes them, PCORTF can rollover unused funds, which provides a chance to conduct longer-range strategic planning. AHRQ began this process by pulling together an interdisciplinary group at the staff level from across AHRQ's centers, offices, and divisions. The planning process will create the strategic framework with appropriate stakeholder engagement, invest in the necessary infrastructure to accomplish AHRQ's goals for PCORTF, and then develop an evaluation of its efforts.

Rhodes explained that AHRQ's mission is to "synthesize and support the dissemination of evidence into practice and train the next generation of patient-centered outcomes researchers," with an overarching vision of delivering equitable, whole-person care across the life span (AHRQ, 2022). AHRQ developed a strategic framework with five high-level priorities and desired outcomes for trust fund investments through fiscal year 2029 to fulfill this mission (see Appendix D). The five priority areas of the framework are

1. health equity;
2. prevention and improved care of people with chronic conditions;
3. patient, family, and provider experience of care that enhances trust in the health care system;
4. high-quality, safe care that is aligned with national health priorities; and
5. primary care transformation.

AHRQ published a notice in the *Federal Register* seeking public input that closed a week before this workshop, said Rhodes. AHRQ has also established a subcommittee of the AHRQ National Advisory Committee to address issues pertaining to the strategic framework. In addition, AHRQ is coordinating closely with PCORI and ASPE to tell one narrative of how the three entities spend PCORTF dollars to enhance health care and health care quality. This framework, she noted, will evolve, as will the projects it funds and the national priorities driving those projects.

COMMUNITY HEALTH WORKERS: A LINK BETWEEN PROVIDER AND PATIENT

Shreya Kangovi, founding executive director of the Penn Center for Community Health Workers and associate professor at the University of Pennsylvania Perelman School of Medicine, began by explaining that community health workers[1] (CHWs) embody the concepts of person-centered, equitable, whole-person care across the life span. The nation's 86,000 community-based organizations employ the majority of the nation's CHWs though public health departments and, more recently, value-based health care organizations.[2] Kangovi noted CHWs are not siloed in one part of the care continuum or one specific patient population. They are frontline public health workers with a uniquely broad and deep understanding of the community they serve. This understanding allows them to fulfill roles across and beyond the care continuum, such as:

- providing social and emotional support,
- care navigation and care coordination,

---

[1] A community health worker is a frontline public health worker who uses their trust and/or membership in a community to link community members to social and health-related services. They may also engage in advocacy, health education, or health communication (APHA, 2022).

[2] Value-based health care is a health care delivery model in which providers, including hospitals and physicians, are paid based on patient health outcomes (NEJM Catalyst, 2017).

- cultural mediation,
- life coaching,
- advocacy, and
- outreach.

Kangovi noted that CHWs can address all levels of health inequity. Many people consider health inequity an imbalance of diseases that affect "vulnerable populations," but she pushes back on that notion. She defines health inequity as a psychological condition that starts with people who have privilege, which creates psychological distortions such as savior complex, group narcissism, and implicit bias that influence policy decisions. These decisions often shape the distribution of wealth and power within institutions and across society, she continued. In turn, these societal factors affect living conditions and health-affecting behaviors, such as smoking or a lack of physical activity, and produce disparities across a range of different health conditions and outcomes (Figure 2-1). She noted that adopting this framework for the root causes of health inequities changes the dynamics of who health inequity affects. Health inequity is "a condition that starts in one group of people but whose symptoms are manifest in a different group of people," said Kangovi.

Kangovi explained that CHWs can bridge the gap between individuals and their health care team, and they can also coach individuals on behavior change, such as quitting smoking or getting more exercise. Additionally, beyond directly addressing health concerns, CHWs have lived experience regarding health inequity. This allows them to change the distribution of wealth and power in institutions because they have the power and autonomy to help shape health care interventions and decisions. Kangovi suggested that

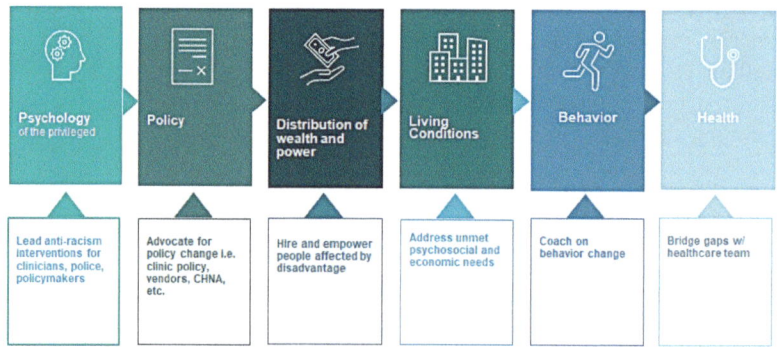

FIGURE 2-1 Community health workers address all stages of health inequity
SOURCE: Presented by Shreya Kangovi on June 9, 2022, at Accelerating the Use of Findings from Patient-Centered Outcomes Research in Clinical Practice to Improve Health and Health Care: A Workshop Series.

CHWs are also some of the best policy advocates she has met, in large part because of their lived experience. She offered an example of her own institution, where executives now have CHWs mentoring them to help foster awareness of their own privilege and to make equitable decisions.

Brea Burke, a Virginia certified CHW with Healing Hands Health Center and founder of CHWUnited, explained that serving the community is something that has been part of her life since she was a young girl. She would often join her father, a pastor, when he visited people in the hospital or at their home. Burke noted that CHWs take on many different roles depending on the needs of their patients: "We become what the patient needs most: a friend, a confidant, a gym partner, a walking buddy, an advocate at appointments, a shoulder to cry on," she said. She described CHWs as the link that helps health care providers see and understand the whole picture of their patients' lives, not just the part they see in their offices.

Burke told the story of one of her clients, a woman whose clinical providers thought might need some extra support, for which they referred her to Burke. When she first met her new client at the client's home, she discovered that the only furniture the woman had was two wooden kitchen chairs and a small wooden table. The woman had disposed of the rest of her furniture due to a previous bed bug infestation in her apartment building and could not afford new furniture. Burke learned during that first conversation that the woman had experienced a cocaine addiction following the loss of her husband, in addition to experiencing an ongoing alcohol use disorder and mental health disorders. Burke helped the woman identify priorities and set goals that would improve her health and happiness. Burke then provided support for the woman to attain those goals, such as connecting her with a community organization to acquire furniture, walking with her to the nearest grocery store, and connecting her to mental health services.

IMPaCT: A Case Study of Translating PCOR to Improve Health

Kangovi explained that she and her colleagues began developing the Individualized Management for Patient-Centered Targets (IMPaCT) program 12 years ago, when she partnered with a CHW from southwest Philadelphia to learn about the health-related concerns of the residents of south and southwest Philadelphia. Specifically, they asked what community members identified as barriers to maintaining good health and what the health care system could be doing differently to address those barriers. They interviewed 1,500 people in a variety of locations, including on their front porches, at their bedsides, and in shelters for people experiencing homelessness. Kangovi noted that the people interviewed lived in chronically under-resourced neighborhoods.

She described three common themes that were observed in the interviews. The first theme was the importance of the social determinants of health, as those real life issues drove their lives. The second theme was that the people interviewed wanted help managing those real life issues from someone to whom they could relate, particularly someone who had similar lived experiences. The third theme was that they wanted to retain power. The people that were interviewed wanted support and resources so they could manage their health. She noted that these themes connected with the work typically done by community health workers.

Kangovi noted that when she began researching the barriers to successful CHW programs, she expected the primary barriers would be lack of funding and political will. However, she learned that the main impediments were implementation factors, staff turnover, lack of infrastructure, not truly understanding what CHWs should be doing, and a lack of understanding of how to incorporate this unique workforce into the health care system without destroying or over medicalizing[3] them.

Kangovi and colleagues developed the IMPaCT program, which was informed by their interviews and her research of the community health worker field. The program includes a stepwise process to recruit, train, and deploy CHWs (Figure 2-2). The program recruits CHWs through community health organizations and emphasizes finding people that have the needed interpersonal skills more than those with formal training. The IMPaCT model includes providing CHWs with a formalized framework to consider who they should be supporting, as well as when to make the connection at a time and place that is useful and comfortable for the patient. The IMPaCT team developed "playbooks" that teach the CHWs how to get to know their clients' life stories and turn that information into person-driven goals that translate into meaningful action. Kangovi and her collaborators also developed best practices for supervisors and developed key performance indicators for program evaluation.

Kangovi said that she and her IMPaCT colleagues have evaluated their CHW program through multiple disease-agnostic, person-centered clinical trials. Inclusion criteria for these studies required the client to

- be a Medicaid or dually eligible beneficiary;
- live in an under-resourced zip code; and
- have had either one hospitalization or two or more chronic conditions, including smoking or obesity.

---

[3] Medicalization refers to the degree to which society considers something to be "medical" in nature, such as by considering a profession to be part of the broader health care system, or a certain condition being considered a disease (Maturo, 2012).

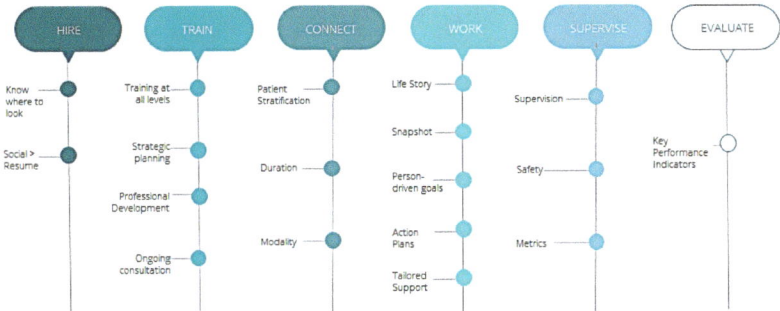

FIGURE 2-2 Project IMPaCT's ordered process that allows community health workers to achieve success consistently
SOURCE: Presented by Shreya Kangovi on June 9, 2022, at Accelerating the Use of Findings from Patient-Centered Outcomes Research in Clinical Practice to Improve Health and Health Care: A Workshop Series.

These studies found that the IMPaCT program approach to CHWs produced net savings on health care spending of $2,500 per person per year (Kangovi et al., 2020; Morgan et al., 2016). They also found that patients supported by CHWs had fewer days of hospitalization when compared to matched control patients who did not have support from a CHW (Vasan et al., 2020). Those clients also had higher scores on health care services surveys regarding primary care access and quality, and also had improved chronic disease management and mental health (Kangovi, 2018).

Kangovi noted that the IMPaCT team has also translated and disseminated some of its work to inform public policy. For example, President Biden included Medicare coverage for CHWs in the fiscal year (FY) 2023 budget proposal. In January 2022, a bipartisan group of senators introduced the Building a Sustainable Workforce for Healthy Communities Act.[4] This bill would reauthorize and revise a Centers for Disease Control and Prevention (CDC) program that supports the use of CHWs to improve health outcomes in medically underserved communities. In April 2022, the Health Resources and Services Administration (HRSA) announced it would provide $226.5 million to launch a multiyear CHW training program.[5]

---

[4] *Building a Sustainable Workforce for Healthy Communities Act*, S.3479, 117th Cong, 2nd sess. (January 11, 2022).
[5] Additional information is available at https://www.hhs.gov/about/news/2022/04/15/hhs-announces-226-million-launch-community-health-worker-training-program.html (accessed September 15, 2022).

DISCUSSION

Hughes opened the discussion by asking Kangovi to list what she considers the top barriers to implementing CHWs more broadly in U.S. health care systems. Kangovi replied that the barriers have changed over the years. When she first started IMPaCT, the primary barrier was a lack of evidence to inform how to best disseminate and implement these programs. However, there have now been dozens of randomized, controlled trials conducted across the country and internationally that consistently point to a set of best practices for implementation. These best practices have been outlined in reports from the National Committee for Quality Assurance and the World Health Organization, among others (Lau et al, 2021; WHO, 2018b). She emphasized that it is important to understand that training is not the only necessity to produce good outcomes.

Kangovi highlighted two funding related challenges for CHW programs that should be addressed at the policy level. First, she said, there is a need for sustainable and adequate funding for CHW programs, as opposed to the current patchwork of grants and demonstration projects. She called for Medicaid and Medicare to cover the full range of evidence-based support provided by CHWs. Second, she said, funding for CHW programs should be tied to implementing best practices, and regulation is needed to protect the professional identity of this workforce and ensure the quality of the services they provide. Burke echoed these concerns, noting that her position is currently funded by a grant.

3

Workshop 1, Session 1: Developing a Coordinated Interdisciplinary Approach to Decision Making around Where to Focus AHRQ's PCORTF Investments

> **Key Messages Presented by Individual Speakers**
>
> - Strategies that may be beneficial to address concerns about trust include adding formal language about building trust through co-creation in partnership agreements, understanding the historical context and root causes of the problem to be studied, laying out a plan for sustainability, and recognizing partners (Gupta)
> - Dissemination of research results must occur beyond academic journals and should be delivered in a form that is useful for the community the research was designed to benefit. (Gupta)
> - Forming community advisory councils early and engaging them frequently in the development, implementation, and dissemination of interventions is critical for the success of any community-based health research program. (Nease)
> - In partnerships, consensus is not required, but ensuring that no one group dominates a process and that everyone involved can see their mark on the final product is essential. (Nease)

Session moderator Catherine Kothari, associate professor and population health scientist in the division of epidemiology and biostatistics at Western Michigan University Homer Stryker MD School of Medicine and senior epidemiologist for Cradle-Kalamazoo, began the session by highlighting several concepts. Interdisciplinary, she said, refers to the various clinical and community sectors that touch health care systems and the delivery of health services. This includes the actors within these sectors and the individuals who influence or make medical, administrative, or policy decisions, including the patients themselves. Health equity, she continued, refers to more than just equal access; it includes reaching people where they are with respectful and responsive care and services. Finally, she described engagement as going beyond having a conversation to understanding each other's perspectives and adapting behaviors and practices to meet each other's priorities more effectively.

A FOCUS ON GOALS AND AUTHENTIC PARTNERSHIPS

Reshma Gupta, chief of population health and accountable care at University of California Davis Health, a member of the University of California Health's population health steering body, and co-director of Costs of Care, Inc., began her presentation by noting her positions as a practicing internist, trained health services researcher, and a member of the population health leadership team across all University of California Health campuses. Through these roles, she has experienced all sides of the challenges that investigators face when trying to engage key partners in patient-centered outcomes research (PCOR). These challenges include bridging interdisciplinary silos and the need for authentic community, health system, and organizational engagement.

Gupta said that an important lesson she has learned more from her experiences as a manager rather than as a researcher is that it is important to understand who the key partners are, what matters most to them, what the likely friction points between key partners are, and what strategies will mitigate those friction points. Ultimately, she said, co-creation[1] and human-centered design[2] help provide answers to those questions. She identified the following as key partners in PCOR:

---

[1] Co-creation refers to involving community members or other relevant stakeholders throughout the research process, from study design to dissemination of the results (Stock et al., 2021).

[2] Human-centered design is a process and a set of techniques used to create new solutions for the world. Solutions include products, services, environments, organizations, and modes of interaction. The reason this process is called "human-centered" is because it starts with the people we are designing for (Göttgens and Oertelt-Prigione, 2021).

- patients and families;
- community members and community leaders;
- clinical specialists, nurses, and pharmacists;
- occupational, respiratory, and speech therapists;
- care managers and navigators, community health workers, social workers, and goal-of-care extenders;
- mental health counselors;
- financial counselors;
- health care delivery system representatives with a special focus on community health and safety-net facilities to ensure that equity is considered;
- social science specialists, such as economists; and
- representatives of rural health, state, and public health directors.

She noted that the opportunity exists for the Agency for Healthcare Research and Quality (AHRQ) to cocreate strategies for improved fund allocation through advisory structures that include community partners. Their input can help guide AHRQ's investments to improve alignment between investigators and partners.

Gupta said that building trust plays an important role in reducing points of friction. Partners may be concerned that their input may not be fully incorporated. This can lead to missed targets on implementation, limited results, adversely affected relationships, and a lack of a sustainable plan. Another area in which trust plays a role in reducing points of friction is related to relationships. Trust must be developed between the investigators and the community-based organization (CBO) so that the CBO can feel confident the research process will not compromise the relationships that the organization relies on to do its work. Gupta explained that for a study to impact the community, health system, or partner organizations, investigators must grasp the historical context and root causes of the problem they are trying to address before they jump to developing solutions.

She noted that misalignment between researchers' proposed study population and the focus areas of CBOs can also create challenges. For example, some individuals in the community may have health issues that are too complex to be included in a given study, or the study's exclusion criteria may be too broad to include certain community members. Community partners, she continued, may want the scope of the research to increase so that the intervention can benefit a larger share of their constituents. In addition, the leaders of some organizations may themselves want to benefit from the research by way of recognition or other means when the resulting intervention is disseminated.

Gupta emphasized that authentic engagement with the community, health system, or organization is paramount to understand what matters to these partners. These groups want to ensure that engagement is not being conducted only for the purpose of completing a study requirement. Gupta explained that while there is no one type of partner, other common desires include

- Feeling understood about the external and internal pressures, outcomes, resources, challenges, and strengths they have;
- Staying aligned with patient, community, or organizational goals and strategic plans;
- Co-creating plans through a process of coming to understand the problem, discovery, potential solutions, interventions, dissemination, and communication together; and
- Recognizing that they are doing much of the hard work and that implementation opens vital relationships they have with their own staff or their partners to the investigators.

Gupta offered ideas for how a flexible strategic approach might relieve common friction points. Strategies that may be beneficial to address concerns about trust include adding formal language about building trust through co-creation in partnership agreements, understanding the historical context and root causes of the problem to be studied, laying out a plan for sustainability, and recognizing partners. Moreover, Gupta suggested the example of including time for researchers to understand the community's current state and root causes of the problem to be studied. It could also be helpful to include a qualitative component to help address concerns around real-world effects of these interventions, Gupta added.

PRACTICE-BASED RESEARCH NETWORKS AND COMMUNITY ENGAGEMENT

Donald Nease, professor of family medicine and the Green-Edelman Chair for practice-based research at the University of Colorado Anschutz Medical Campus, spoke from the perspective of someone who has led several research infrastructures at his institution. Such programs include the community engagement infrastructure that is part of the Colorado Clinical and Translational Sciences Institute (CCTSI) and the State Networks of Colorado Ambulatory Practices and Partners (SNOCAP) practice-based research networks (PBRNs), of which there are five in Colorado.

Nease explained that community and patient advisory group members are involved throughout the entire research process. For example, one of the PBRNs recently completed a survey of practices that one of the patient advisory groups suggested because it was interested in learning how clinician and staff burnout affects care from the patient's perspective. The advisory group helped design questions that the PBRN distributed to practices to identify the signs of burnout that patients observe. Advisory group members also copresent and coauthor presentations and papers and are involved in the local dissemination of a study's findings. Nease said that what the advisory council members say when presenting about a research project is often more compelling than what the research team says. In addition, patient and community advisory groups can serve as consultants to other groups around the country or coinvestigators on other projects.

Nease said one of the ways in which CCTSI facilitates local uptake and use of evidence is through an approach it calls community or boot camp translation. This approach began with a project funded by the Centers for Disease Control and Prevention focused on increasing colorectal cancer screening rates in rural eastern Colorado. CCTSI partnered with the High Plains Research Network's community advisory council and brought an expert in colorectal cancer to one of its meetings. Council members had the opportunity to ask questions and interact with an endoscopy simulator to better understand the procedure. That hands-on opportunity led the council members to realize that colonoscopies are a preventive procedure that can remove precancerous polyps before they develop into full-blown cancer. At that meeting the council members asked if it was possible to call the procedure something other than colorectal cancer screening. The resulting discussion led to a shift in the language to make it more relevant for that community.

Nease noted that both the SNOCAP and CCTSI infrastructures share several core principles, the first of which is that while facts may be universal, implementation is local. For example, while colorectal cancer screening can save lives, communicating that message effectively so that people get screened often requires an understanding of the needs and priorities of the local community. In that regard, co-creation is an important part of the programs he oversees.

The second core principle is "Nothing for us, without us," which Nease said means working with community members from the very beginning of a project. The third core principle is that outreach *begins* with an answer, while engagement *ends* with one. He noted that often in academics, outreach occurs in the form of bringing answers to a community without first engaging with that community to learn their questions, which at times can be an effective approach. However, bidirectional learning that ends with an answer can better fit the purpose and interests of a particular community.

In closing, Nease listed questions that he and his colleagues ask themselves regularly to ensure effective and equitable community engagement:

- Do we have the right people at the table who can provide a perspective from their lived experiences, and do they include those who would be affected by such a project?

- Are we engaging people equitably, and have we lowered all the barriers to hearing their voices through actions such as holding meetings at times convenient for the community rather than for the researchers or by providing child care?
- Is our work building capacity and will our participants be able to carry this experience to other kinds of work?

DISCUSSION

Considering Opportunities for Professional Education

Kothari opened the discussion with a question from a workshop participant, who asked Nease and Gupta to discuss how the work they are doing could be translated to efforts directed toward influencing medical school curricula and to shift the emphasis from specialization toward community-engaged primary care. Nease replied that his institution has a tradition called mentored student activity for its medical students, and one option is for students to work with faculty who are engaged in community work. One project, called Colorado Students Against Racism in Medicine, has continued longitudinally through several successive groups of medical students. The success of those programs recently led his institution to redesign its medical school curriculum to include community engagement and ensure that all students have a community engagement experience that spans the 4 years of medical school.

Gupta said that the University of California's medical schools have a number of programs focused on community-engaged primary care. Some programs, courses, and electives link students to community engagement outreach efforts focused on communities affected by health care disparities or those with social needs. She said that medical schools are also starting to integrate the idea of co-creation into coursework.

Considering Partner Relationships

The next questioner asked Nease if he encountered challenges with whether community members that were asked to participate in advisory groups felt comfortable in that role. He replied that he is frequently asked how he recruits community partners. His answer is that community members tend to care about what is going on in their community regarding health care, so they usually welcome the opportunity to participate in an advisory group. He acknowledged that when a community translation effort first starts, there is some of the aforementioned concern among the participants, so he and his colleagues spend time in the initial meeting building a sense of belonging and community within the group. This helps ensure that everyone feels they can share their perspective freely.

Kothari then asked the two panelists if they could describe a situation where partners had competing interests. Gupta replied that she has many examples of this challenge. One example involves a study around equity in lung cancer screening. While everyone was motivated to move this project forward and increase its scale quickly, health care systems across the nation are short of staff to work on new initiatives. As an administrator, she has to deal with the challenges of prioritizing multiple initiatives running simultaneously, while as a researcher, she wants her project to be at the top of the prioritization list. The key to resolving conflicts and competing interests, she said, is to have honest conversations built on trust among the partners and to put in the hard work needed to find a solution. Nease explained that the process of collaborating with research partners is not necessarily about reaching consensus, but it is to ensure that no one group dominates the process and everyone involved can see their effect on the final product.

Kothari asked Gupta if she could speak from her perspective and experience about whether there are points in the dissemination and implementation of research findings where she finds it most critical to engage partners and if so, if there are specific partners that are critical to engage at specific points in the research process. Gupta answered that when she works with her program's fellows, she emphasizes that academic publication is not sufficient for dissemination. The research team is often not the right group to deliver key messages. It is important for community partners to play a significant role in dissemination because they have insight into how best to deliver information in a manner that will be useful to the community.

4

Workshop 1, Session 2: Training PCOR Investigators

> **Key Messages Presented by Individual Speakers**
> - PCOR researcher training that includes stakeholders at community health centers increases opportunities for research that is informed by the needs of the community. (Mohanty)
> - It is helpful to understand and recognize the power dynamics informed by historical and present-day opportunity differentials that have disproportionately impacted specific communities when conducting PCOR. (Gonzalez)
> - PCOR researchers can gain important insight by ensuring active participation by those who are affected by the issues that research is meant to address. (Gonzalez)
> - Practice cultural humility and power-sharing when working with the community on any research project. (Gonzalez)

COLLABORATIONS FOR TRAINING COMMUNITY-BASED RESEARCHERS

Nivedita Mohanty, chief research officer and director of evidence-based practice at AllianceChicago and clinical associate professor at the Feinberg School of Medicine, discussed examples of patient-centered outcomes research

(PCOR) training programs for community health center staff. She began by describing the Collaborations for Health and Empowered Community-Based Scientists (CHECS) program. CHECS is a training and mentorship program for community health centers run by AllianceChicago.[1] AllianceChicago is a network of community health centers across the nation for which Mohanty's organization provides technology infrastructure, a clinical collaboration infrastructure, and a structure for practice-based research. The 72 safety-net organizations in the network serve over 3.6 million patients at over 400 sites of care delivery in 19 states. AllianceChicago has a mission of improving personal, community, and public health through innovative collaboration. Mohanty noted that community health centers are committed to whole-person care, which is why it is important that PCOR researcher training includes members of the community health center workforce in advancing patient-centered outcomes research.

Mohanty explained that community health centers are the largest source of primary preventive care for the nation's medically underserved adults and children. These organizations provide care for 1 in 9 children, 1 in 3 people with incomes at or below the federal poverty level, 1 in 5 residents of rural communities, and nearly 377,000 veterans. Mohanty said approximately 29 million people nationwide rely on a Health Resources and Services Administration (HRSA)-supported community health center for affordable, accessible primary care. She noted that PCOR research questions often originate outside of community health centers, which is something she designed CHECS to change.

Mohanty described an experience she had when she was a full-time pediatrician that inspired her interest in research. She was having difficulty drawing blood to screen for jaundice from a first-time mother's newborn child. The mother asked her why she was not using the transcutaneous device that was commonly used in hospitals to screen for jaundice. One of the reasons her clinic had not implemented that tool was it had not been tested extensively in primary care, particularly among children of color, who were the majority her clinic's patients. She was able to procure seed funding to explore the reliability of the transcutaneous device in her setting because of her faculty position at a nearby university. This research produced findings that resulted in a change in practice to use the transcutaneous device to test bilirubin in her clinic.

She noted that in her role at AllianceChicago, she has learned that not every practitioner has the same opportunity to conduct research to answer questions they might have. The CHECS program is intended to address that. CHECS helps her organization's stakeholders obtain experience in PCOR through a Eugene Washington Patient-Centered Outcomes Research Institute (PCORI) Engagement Award. This allows community health practitio-

---

[1] Additional information is available at https://alliancechicago.org (accessed July 17, 2022).

ners to cultivate ideas that their experiences, patients, and communities have informed in partnership with academic researchers and then pursue funding to implement their research ideas.

Mohanty explained CHECS participation has several benefits including

- obtaining PCOR skills and knowledge;
- support to investigate ideas for improving primary care services and patient outcomes in community health;
- support and mentorship from experienced PCOR researchers;
- continuing education opportunities; and
- opportunities for peer-to-peer learning and development of partnerships across community health centers.

The CHECS program's success relies on developing capacity to support community health center investigators to build research skills to explore research ideas and helping those investigators learn how to engage teams to implement their research and further define their questions. One of the CHECS program goals is that participants who complete the program will be able to pursue funding, either alone or with a partner, to research their ideas in the context of community health centers.

The CHECS program is an online, self-directed learning curriculum that AllianceChicago offers in conjunction with partners in the Clinical Directors Network, a nonprofit, practice-based research network and clinician training organization. It uses the Enhancing Community Health Center Patient-Centered Outcomes Research Engagement (EnCoRE) online training program. EnCoRE allows people to view trainings in a self-directed manner and receive continuing education credits at no cost. Mohanty and her colleagues developed a series of training webcasts based on feedback from Alliance Chicago's health center partners about training needs to conduct PCOR.

AllianceChicago recently conducted a 12-month, intensive mentored PCOR training fellowship program. Mohanty explained that funding for the fellowship program supported in-person travel for training sessions, salary support for protected time for the fellows, and an honorarium for the mentors that supported the fellows throughout their projects. Training topics included PCOR, how to engage patients with lived experience, community-based participatory research, research collaboration, using clinical data for research, research dissemination, grant review, and mindfulness self-coaching. Fellows had a variety of roles at community health centers, such as medical assistants, nurse practitioners, and chief medical officers. The fellows collaborated with their mentors on projects relevant to community health. Mohanty added that the program was also fortunate to work with academic partners who were generous with their time. Participants valued the pragmatic and hands-on skills they developed, particularly regarding stakeholder engagement, the intersection of quality improvement and research, basic research methods and study design, fundamentals of statistics, and how to achieve high-impact dissemination other than through peer-reviewed publication.

Mohanty described several observations and lessons learned from her organization's experience with the fellowship program. The mentorship component of the program created valuable opportunities for bidirectional learning. Two important lessons were that learning flowed bidirectionally between fellows and mentors and that competing priorities at community health centers are pervasive. PCOR investigators outside of the traditional academic setting find it challenging to procure seed or research funding. The program also highlighted some specific facilitators of success. Those include

- providing structured and protected time for PCOR training,
- ensuring fellows and mentors have aligned interests,
- engaging in multimodal communication with patients involved in research,
- opportunities for peer interaction, and
- buy-in from community health center leadership.

Mohanty noted that three projects that were developed in the fellowship program received implementation funding. Eighty-eight percent of the fellows reported that the in-person trainings strengthened their skills and the overall project, and 92 percent said that mentorship strengthened their skills and the overall project. She noted that all of the organizations that participated in CHECS have since engaged in multiple research studies and collaborations. Mohanty added that AllianceChicago continues to offer opportunities to build partnerships, PCOR training, and capacity-building opportunities.

EDUCATIONAL TRAINING FOR THE NEXT GENERATION OF INVESTIGATORS

Cynthia Gonzalez, director of the Pardee RAND Graduate School's Community-Partnered Policy and Action Stream Ph.D. program in policy analysis and assistant professor at Charles R. Drew University of Medicine and Science, discussed equity-centered collaborations that went beyond traditional systems of training PCOR investigators. She began by noting that her identity as "a first-generation Chicana from Watts, an inner-city neighborhood in Los Angeles" has informed her work. She explained that in order for her to understand health disparities and inequities, she had to become a student of her own community. That effort led to her interest in participatory community engagement, place-based health, and community partnerships. Gonzalez described several of Charles R. Drew University of Medicine and Science's (CDU's) collaboration programs. CDU is located in Los Angeles County and was founded with a commitment to cultivating diverse health professional leaders who are dedicated to social justice and health equity for underserved populations through outstanding education, research, clinical service, and community engagement.

CDU's core curricular experience, the CDU Advantage,[2] has a social justice focus that includes local and global perspectives. Gonzalez explained that CDU's strong health disparities research portfolio enables students to engage in research through specific focus areas that are relevant to the communities that surround the university. CDU has incorporated various engagement models as part of its curricular activities to help ensure applied learning. One such model is the community faculty track.[3] This is a unique pedagogical approach to academic-community partnerships that recruits local resident community experts affiliated with a community of interest or a nonprofit agency to serve as faculty in the College of Medicine, similar to clinical faculty. The community faculty members offer critical expertise that emphasizes the importance of understanding both community and academic perspectives to improve a community's health. They teach courses that introduce students to critical social issues, the principles of community engagement, and capacity building in community health, public health, place-based health, organizational development, social justice, equity, and civil rights. Community faculty also collaborate with CDU researchers as co-investigators, serve as principal investigators for their own research projects, and participate in the admissions review process for medical school applicants. In addition, community faculty support knowledge dissemination by planning local conferences, presenting their work at local and national conferences, and sitting on university committees, including institutional review boards.

The Pardee RAND Graduate School,[4] where Gonzalez serves as the director of the community-partnered policy and action stream, is a multidisciplinary graduate program focused on policy analysis and the ways in which policy analysis shapes society that also offers a full-time Ph.D. program. Students at Pardee RAND apply to one of three engagement streams: research, analysis, and design; technology applications and implications; and community-partnered policy and action, which is the stream Gonzalez leads. The expectation for

---

[2] Additional information is available at https://www.cdrewu.edu/COM/PMA/CDU Advantage (accessed September 14, 2022).

[3] Additional information available at https://www.cdrewu.edu/research/Center/Community (accessed September 14, 2022).

[4] Additional information is available at https://www.prgs.edu (accessed July 17, 2022).

this third stream is that it will merge academic and applied work, training students to bring their research into action and implementation. The focus of this stream is two-fold: develop and train the next generation of innovative thinkers, and do so by working with community partners to effect change. Coursework includes learning about intersectionality, engaging communities in research, mixed methods research, and dissemination and implementation science.[5] Students are required to have a community partner as an external member of their dissertation committee. Students develop interpersonal skills including how to practice cultural humility, engage in deep listening, and work to understand multiple perspectives and experiences relevant to the history of the communities that they aim to serve. Gonzalez explained that the entire learning experience emphasizes valuing community knowledge and building relationships with those partners to produce sustainable change. She said the holistic curriculum exposes and prepares students to be future scholars who are mindful of how social dynamics affect research.

Gonzalez then spoke about the Watts Rising Collaborative,[6] a partnership between Watts residents, more than 50 cross-sector organizations led by the Los Angeles Housing Authority, the Los Angeles mayor's office, and the local city council district. In 2019, the collaborative received a grant from the state of California to fund 24 community-identified infrastructure projects. These projects were designed to combine data-informed decisions and community engagement to develop strategies to reduce greenhouse gas emissions, promote economic development, improve public health, engage community, and avoid displacement through data-informed decisions and community engagement. The Watts Rising Collaborative partnered with investigators to assist in data collection through neighborhood assessments. This included interviews and focus groups to help investigators understand community reach, priorities, assets, and needs, as well as to ensure that projects produced meaningful change in public and environmental health outcomes.

Gonzalez noted the Watts Rising Collaborative also offers opportunities for students from middle school to graduate school to participate in projects. The collaborative has also created a structure that enables community-academic partnerships and immersive training that incorporates equity-minded approaches. She added that these activities enable collaborations that break down silos, engage and involve the community, and allow researchers to gain a

---

[5] Dissemination and Implementation Science (DIS) is a growing research field that seeks to inform how evidence-based interventions can be successfully adopted, implemented, and maintained in health care delivery and community settings (Holtrop et al., 2018).

[6] Additional information is available at https://www.wattsrising.org (accessed September 14, 2022).

greater understanding of the priorities of people in communities of color and communities that have been historically marginalized and isolated.

Gonzalez concluded her presentation by sharing lessons she has learned from her experiences with the projects she discussed. Those lessons included the following:

- It is critical to understand and recognize that power dynamics informed by historical and present-day opportunity differentials have disproportionately impacted specific communities.
- People affected by the issues that a research project is designed to address should be included in the project as active participants with valuable expertise and insight.
- There is a need for collaboration across disciplines and sectors while also engaging with and learning from the community.
- PCOR researchers should seek opportunities to include community-based participatory research methods and qualitative and mixed methods into research models.

She explained that qualitative and mixed methods research add a narrative to the metrics that provide a deeper understanding of what factors most affect a community and how it responds to challenges.

DISCUSSION

Session moderator Meghan Lane-Fall, vice chair of inclusion, diversity, and equity; the David E. Longnecker associate professor of anesthesiology and critical care; and associate professor of biostatistics, epidemiology, and informatics at the University of Pennsylvania Perelman School of Medicine, led the discussion.

Research and Quality Improvement

Lane-Fall asked Mohanty to speak about how she conceptualizes quality improvement and research and the relationship between the two. Mohanty replied that quality improvement and research both play a critical role in improving patient care and the function of health care systems. She opined that community health centers may have less difficulty conceptualizing quality improvement because they have a built-in infrastructure for it as part of clinical care and can implement change fairly rapidly. Research typically involves more structured protocols, has more regulatory components to consider, and usually is more time intensive. She explained that the goal of research is to produce findings or evidence that might be generalizable, whereas quality improvement focuses on things that may be more relevant on a local scale.

Future Training Investments

Lane-Fall asked Gonzalez to discuss what Agency for Healthcare Research and Quality (AHRQ) should consider when making future investments in training PCOR investigators. Gonzalez replied that AHRQ should consider opportunities to bridge the applied research setting and academic research setting in a manner that effectively engages the strengths of both settings. She also highlighted that researchers would benefit from engaging with the communities that they seek to study to gain insight that will inform more effective research questions. Mohanty suggested that future PCOR training investments should include community-based research. She also suggested including requirements for thoughtful integration of community members during the planning process or developing partnerships with community organizations in future funding opportunities.

CDU's Community Faculty Model

Lane-Fall asked Gonzalez to further discuss CDU's community faculty model, including any insights around how it has been received by stakeholders. Gonzalez explained that the community faculty model stems from a partnership between an academic researcher, the late Dr. Loretta Jones, and an exceptional community in South Central Los Angeles. Jones recognized that there were people in communities, which she referred to as the Ph.D.s of the sidewalk, whose expertise in health equity and community engagement was just as relevant as that of academic scholars and aligned well with the university's mission and values. This led to creation of CDU's community faculty model. CDU also established a division of community engagement that identifies community leaders who might be interested in becoming a community faculty member.

Sustaining Community Based PCOR

Lane-Fall then asked the panelists to discuss approaches for developing sustainable community-based PCOR projects. Mohanty replied that her organization has had some opportunities that enable them to build sustainable infrastructure through funds from federal grants and suggested that funding to support infrastructure development rather than specific projects might help improve sustainability. She noted that while the duration of the funding was limited, the resulting infrastructure remains, including committees that meet monthly to evaluate research projects for their potential benefits to the community. She noted that it is also important for researchers to educate organization leadership about the benefits of their program in order to garner the institutional support necessary for sustainability.

Gonzalez agreed that infrastructure investment can benefit sustainability, noting that while the community faculty program started with a grant, it now is embedded in courses, admissions reviews, and partnerships with other academic institutions. However, the Watts Rising Collaborative continues to rely primarily on grant funding for its work, which creates challenges around building sustainability into some projects.

Identifying and Balancing Priorities

An audience member asked Gonzalez to discuss how she prioritizes which community issues to focus on in her various roles and how that reflects her relationships and level of trust with certain communities. Gonzalez replied that she is passionate about working in Watts because members of her family live there and her work can help improve the quality of their lives. She added that in her work, she tries to focus on community assets as much as on needs or deficits and on priorities set by the community. Gonzalez noted that this approach requires cultural humility, adding, "We cannot assume that we know what communities are experiencing. We have to ask." She explained that she considers her work in academic institutions training future health care and policy professionals as capacity building. Those future professionals will be prepared to focus on solving the issues that are significantly impacting certain communities while centering social issues such as discrimination and inequity.

Lane-Fall commented that she struggles as a program director to balance the excitement of her trainees about a project and the needs of the system in which they are embedded. Mohanty agreed that this is challenging, and noted she tries to consider where priorities align. Mohanty explained that in her organization's community health centers, alignment occurs with ideas and projects around quality initiatives where two different priorities can work synergistically and where there can be opportunities for collaboration.

Gonzalez said that the academic institutions she works for are seeing a more diverse set of students enter their programs. She noted this includes more students of color, more students who are parents, more first-generation students, and more students with backgrounds of economic insecurity. She explained that while increased student diversity is beneficial, that diversity is accompanied by a greater diversity of lived experiences and research interests. She noted that while PCOR training programs should embrace students' diverse passions, skill building remains essential and balancing the two can be challenging. She described a learning opportunity that developed around an initial conflict between the research interests of a student collaborative and the needs of the grant, and the priorities of the community they were serving. She recounted how one of the collaborative's priorities was to reduce greenhouse gas emissions, in part by planting trees in a community that had very few trees. However, the community they had partnered with wanted jobs, not trees. The solution was to connect greenhouse gas reduction with workforce development, by training residents for jobs in the green industry, such as solar panel installers.

5

Workshop 1, Session 3: Sustainable Strategies and Digital Tools to Expand Implementation of PCOR Findings

> **Key Messages Presented by Individual Speakers**
>
> - A learning collaborative[1] approach can lead to enhanced patient engagement in care; sustained practice transformation; and significant cost reduction. (Schuster)
> - Digital tools can support improved communication between patients and their providers. (Krishnamurti)
> - Digital tools should be designed to support contextually relevant care that matches patient needs and matches clinician workflows through pragmatic designs. (Graham)

USING THE LEARNING COLLABORATIVE APPROACH FOR IMPLEMENTING AND SCALING INNOVATION

James Schuster, chief medical officer for the University of Pittsburgh Medical Center's (UPMC) insurance services division and a member of the

---

[1] A Learning Collaborative is a systematic approach to process improvement based on the Institute for Healthcare Improvement Breakthrough Series Collaborative model. During the Collaborative, organizations will test and implement system changes and measure their impact. They will share their experiences to accelerate learning and broader implementation of best practices (CIBHS, 2015).

PCORI Board of Governors, began by discussing the Community Care Behavioral Health Organization. This is the umbrella organization under which he conducted his work and a subsidiary of UPMC that manages behavioral health services on behalf of over a million Medicaid members across 43 counties in Pennsylvania. Community Care's mission is to improve the health and well-being of the community through the delivery of effective, cost-efficient, and accessible behavioral health services. His work has focused on adults living with serious mental illness. He explained that these individuals frequently have unmet medical needs, placing them at significant risk of developing serious physical health issues (Afzal et al., 2021; De Hert et al., 2009; Rossom et al., 2022). Individuals with serious mental illness die as much as 10 to 20 years younger than the general population because of the increased prevalence of cardiovascular disease, diabetes, and obesity (WHO, 2018a).

Wellness coaching plays a central role in the Behavioral Health Home Plus model developed by Schuster and his colleagues in 2010. Schuster explained that wellness coaching is a strategy for care managers, peer specialists, and other health care staff to help individuals develop skills for self-managing their physical health conditions and other challenges they may face (Swarbrick, 1997, 2006; Zechner et al., 2021). The Behavioral Health Home Plus model focuses on enhancing behavioral health providers' capacity to serve as health homes; to provide comprehensive care management, care coordination and health promotion; and to link service users to community resources. After observing positive results in a small demonstration project, Schuster and colleagues in the UPMC Center for High-Value Health Care conducted a 2-year trial at 11 community mental health settings that treat Medicaid beneficiaries, comparing a provider-directed intervention with this self-management approach (Schuster et al., 2019). The first year of the trial focused on implementation of the model using the Institute for Healthcare Improvement's Learning Collaborative model. Key outcomes from the 2-year trial included

- enhanced patient activation and engagement in care,
- a shift of care from the hospital to community settings,
- sustained practice transformation,
- a greater than 20 percent reduction in cost of care, and
- a cultural change in community care settings that led providers to be more attentive to their own health.

The success of the learning collaborative approach, said Schuster, relies heavily on significant technical support for providers and the agencies that employ them. It is not enough to educate providers or provide tools, said

Schuster. "It is optimal to provide ongoing, structured technical assistance," which the implementation team did over the entire 2-year period, but especially over the first year. For example, the team held two to three learning, engagement, and work review sessions with individual providers each month using a plan-do-study-act (PDSA) approach. Given this success, Schuster and his colleagues expanded the model to new populations using the same learning collaborative approach, including mental health services for adults in community-based settings, in children's outpatient services settings, and in a health home model that uses community- and school-based teams of clinicians to work with children in school, at home, and in other community settings. They also expanded the program to specialty peer support programs, opioid treatment providers, and psychiatric residential treatment providers.

Schuster explained that one key factor that contributed to the success of this implementation effort was the extensive outreach to agency leadership he and his colleagues conducted prior to trying to engage the treatment team. As a result, agency leadership helped drive staff engagement and participation. Qualitative evaluations revealed that providers felt positively about the support and resources they received. Providers also identified areas for improvement, which included further tailoring materials for the youth population, bolstering support for site leadership, and increasing workbook navigation training. Quantitative results showed that the learning collaborative approach increased staff confidence, documented reciprocal communication between behavioral and physical health providers, boosted the number of individuals with a wellness plan, and led to individuals feeling engaged in their own care.

In closing, Schuster said that UPMC's Community Care Behavioral Health Organization is now using the learning collaborative model to address additional practice challenges in other care settings. While he sees this as a successful model, he acknowledged that it does require a significant focus by the agency that is trying to encourage behavior change and the provision of substantial resources to the agencies.

Key facilitators of success include:

1. taking a structured approach to scaling;
2. getting leadership support and participation in the quality improvement team;
3. defining and monitoring key milestones and process and outcome measures;
4. using the PDSA cycle;
5. employing shared learning in a safe and supportive environment; and
6. celebrating successes.

PERSON-CENTERED AND SUSTAINABLE DIGITAL REPRODUCTIVE HEALTH INTERVENTIONS

Tamar Krishnamurti is an assistant professor of medicine and clinical and translational science at the University of Pittsburgh and founder of the FemTech Collaborative within the University of Pittsburgh's Center for Innovative Research on Gender Health Equity. She began by explaining the FemTech Collaborative developed as a result of various researchers' efforts to generate technologies that could supplement the formal health care system to address the goal of improving people's reproductive health and advancing their reproductive health equity.

Krishnamurti opined that reproductive health indexes in the United States, particularly those related to maternal health, are substandard. She said these indexes in part reflect the inequities among people of color and those with preexisting medical conditions. Current health care delivery models can perpetuate poor reproductive health outcomes when they fail to identify people's reproductive risks, their needs, and their preferences. She said current health care delivery models frequently do not adequately support people's autonomy regarding their health care decision-making and inadequately address preventable adverse outcomes in a patient-centered manner.

One of the collaborative's projects was to develop and implement the MyHealthyPregnancy app, which offers early identification and intervention on modifiable pregnancy-related risks. Krishnamurti and her collaborators originally designed the MyHealthyPregnancy platform 6 years ago as a means of identifying and intervening in modifiable risks that are precursors for preterm births prior to 37 weeks of gestation (Krishnamurti et al., 2022). They built the platform in collaboration with behavioral scientists, pregnant individuals, new mothers, physicians, human-computer interaction specialists, and community leaders. An individual's doctor prescribes the app at the first prenatal visit, and the pregnant person uses it to routinely enter information that enables risk factor modeling with a machine learning algorithm and clinical best practice screening. The backend of the system then generates real-time tailored feedback on the individual's pregnancy and provides connections to vetted, patient-centered resources both inside the health care system and in the community. The platform then transfers this information to the health system's physician portal to alert providers and recommend clinical actions for risks that the app detects.

In an 18-month trial of MyHealthyPregnancy that enrolled 7,000 pregnant patients from UPMC's health care system, the FemTech team assessed how well the system detected preeclampsia risk, a leading preventable cause of maternal mortality (Ananth et al., 2013; Ghulmiyyah and Sibai, 2012).

The FemTech team embedded multiple choice questions in the app to assess risk criteria for preeclampsia and to allow the team to determine whether the MyHealthyPregnancy app could facilitate preventive care in the form of aspirin for preeclampsia. Krishnamurti explained that low dose daily aspirin is an evidence based therapy for reducing the risk of preeclampsia (Askie et al., 2007; Xu et al., 2015). They then sent a question out via the app to 2,500 app users to see if their providers had prescribed aspirin and, if so, how often the app users were taking it (Krishnamurti et al., 2021b). Of the 124 individuals at highest risk for preeclampsia, 73 percent had a recommendation for aspirin use in their chart, but only 37 percent were aware of that recommendation. Only about half those who were aware of the recommendation adhered to the prescribed regimen. She said that the study results suggest that the risk criteria for preeclampsia are underused to some extent, and that physicians may have been relying on other cues, such as chronic hypertension, for assessing their patient's risk more heavily than others risk factors. "All of this is to say we were able to use a digital tool like MyHealthyPregnancy to identify risk cues that physicians were relying on and examine which risk factors might be routinely missed," she said. This finding led to a change in clinical practice that UPMC has implemented in its health care system. "This tool let us identify folks at risk from a distance, but it also allowed us to update how they are cared for in person," she said.

Krishnamurti said that when building the MyHealthyPregnancy platform, the FemTech team developed effective predictive machine learning models that allowed the team to pose indirect questions to app users to assess their risk for intimate partner violence throughout pregnancy (Krishnamurti et al., 2021a). She explained that intimate partner violence is a difficult subject to raise with patients. As a result, intimate partner violence often goes undiscussed and undetected. The app has been able to identify pregnant people at risk who were not identified during visits with health care providers. The app connects people identified as at risk with resources. The team has modified that process based on feedback from app users.

Krishnamurti said that two of the most important takeaways from the MyHealthyPregnancy project are that digital tools can sometimes serve as a safe space to disclose sensitive information, and these tools offer a different layer of connection that is particularly important in situations where access to in-person care is limited. She noted the team learned through user feedback, it is important to be mindful of creating tools that feel personalized without being invasive. Another lesson was that the data generated by a digital tool can identify gaps in care, as the app did with preeclampsia. She noted that UPMC's women's health service has done a phenomenal job in combining such data and establishing streamlined responses to risks identified in between routine prenatal care visits.

In terms of the potential for digital women's health tools, Krishnamurti said that the market size for FemTech is estimated to be over a trillion dollars in the next five years, which means the stakes are high for how developers create these technologies and how health systems adopt them. Given that, she shared some additional high-level pitfalls that can arise when technology is seen as an all-encompassing solution rather than as a supplement to care. First, digital tools can create an opportunity for the perpetuation of misinformation as well as for disengagement between patients and health care professionals at a time when human connections are increasingly important for delivering quality care. Second, monetized sensitive data can be used to exploit rather than to alleviate fear. "That is particularly egregious when we know so much about the relationship between stress and poor health outcomes," said Krishnamurti. Third, it is important to remember that machine learning algorithms rely on data that may be inherently biased in how it has been collected and in the modeling assumptions, which can exacerbate inequities. Finally, while smartphone ownership is almost ubiquitous across sociodemographic groups, the quality and the cost of access differs across sociodemographic groups, which can again exacerbate inequities. Given these considerations, the FemTech Collaborative has agreed on the following set of principles to guide how it builds and evaluates its tools (Krishnamurti et al., 2022):

- Ground content in evidence-based science.
- Advance health equity.
- Center the needs and preferences of those seeking care.
- Support patient autonomy in managing their care.
- Incorporate community stakeholders as partners.
- Be iterative and flexible over time with what is being built.

ENGAGING PEOPLE IN INNOVATIVE DIGITAL INTERVENTIONS

Andrea Graham, clinical psychologist and assistant professor at the Center for Behavioral Intervention Technologies at Northwestern University's Feinberg School of Medicine, discussed engaging people with digital tools. She began by noting that digital health tools have been considered an opportunity to extend provision of health care treatment beyond in-person interactions. However, when digital interventions have moved from research settings to real-world settings, they often have low rates of use and retention among patients, failed integration within systems of care, or failed implementation. Graham said the source of the disconnect is that developers often do not design their interventions for users and the contexts in which health systems implement them. Digital tools need to support contextually relevant care that matches the patients' needs through personalization and precision. These tools also need to use pragmatic design approaches to match clinician workflow. She said human-centered design is a useful strategy to make digital health tools that better engage patients and providers (Graham et al., 2019).

Graham and her colleagues have proposed a model of user experience (Figure 5-1) that applies the experimental therapeutics approach, or the science of behavior change, to consider how a digital tool (in this case a theoretical digital mental health tool) can improve the user experience, and thus improve clinical outcomes for users (Graham et al., 2019). The model focuses on how someone uses the digital tool and how useful it is, asking several questions:

- Does it help them achieve things in their daily lives that they would like to achieve?
- Can they navigate it effectively and easily?
- Can they learn to use it easily?
- Are they satisfied with their experience?

Graham explained that integrating new interventions into existing workflows is challenging, particularly integrating digital tools because the delivery differs by design from in-person services. In part, this challenge exists as a

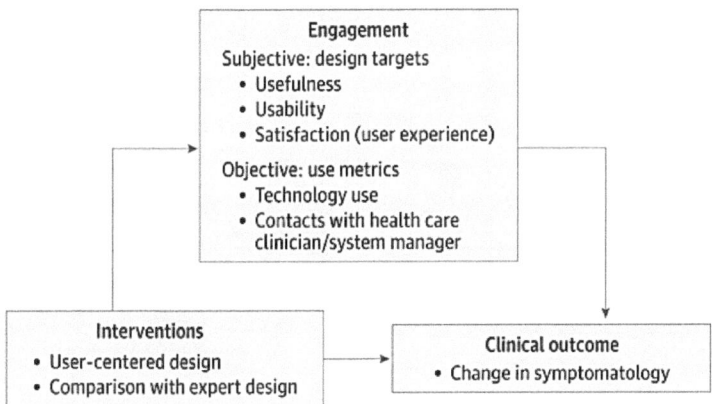

FIGURE 5-1 Conceptual model for experimental therapeutics to target engagement as a mediating mechanism for digital mental health
SOURCE: Reproduced from Graham et al., 2019. Reproduced with permission from JAMA Psychiatry. 2019. 76(12): 1223-1224. Copyright ©2019 American Medical Association. All rights reserved. Presented by Andrea Graham on June 9, 2022, at Accelerating the Use of Findings from Patient-Centered Outcomes Research in Clinical Practice to Improve Health and Health Care: A Workshop Series.

result of the gap in knowing what methods and techniques are most effective for implementing digital interventions into health care settings. Graham and her colleagues assembled a tailored list of implementation strategies specifically for digital health interventions to address that gap (Figure 5-2) (Graham et al., 2019). This list proposes strategies for each phase of implementation. She noted that workflow considerations remain among the least explored but most needed factors toward facilitating implementation of digital health interventions (Torous et al., 2021).

Graham discussed a suite of apps her team has been developing that focus on interventions for depression and anxiety as an example of workflow integration (Graham et al., 2020a). This suite includes digital tools that individuals can use to improve their symptoms and that fit into their daily lives. The suite also provides coaching from a paraprofessional. Graham and her team conducted a clinical trial of the mental health app platform for use in a primary care setting. In terms of workflow integration, specifically referral management, Graham's team deployed several strategies to refer individuals to the app suite (Graham et al., 2020a). Strategies included direct-to-consumer approaches, giving presentations on campus, and clinician referrals through an electronic health record (EHR) alert that would prompt the physician to place an order through the EHR.

Graham explained that one finding from the clinical trial was that interoperability with an EHR is often not consistent, and does not always match what designers think they are trying to build. In this case, EHR referral alone

Proposed Implementation Strategies across Phases of Implementation	
Exploration Phase	
• Conduct needs assessments (e.g., among practitioners, consumers)	• Review DMHI evidence and content
• Align practitioners on DMHI adoption (e.g., consensus discussions)	• Aim to ensure equity in who can access the DMHI
Preparation & Implementation Phases	
• Create a business associate agreement to restrict data usage	• Adopt DMHIs with demonstrated effectiveness
• Determine who is appropriate for the DMHI, and create guidelines	• Design the referral process & inform referring practitioners
• Create and distribute educational materials about the DMHI	• Have "champions" inform consumers about the DMHI
• Be transparent about DMHI data security, privacy, & use	• Be transparent about DMHI requirements, promote autonomy
• Assist with onboarding (e.g., educational materials, point-person)	• Make technical assistance available
• Create and disseminate practice guidelines for delivering the DMHI	• Ensure practitioners are competent to deliver the DMHI
• Offer training & ongoing supervision in using the DMHI	• Monitor practitioners' fidelity to the DMHI protocol
• Specify plans for monitoring & addressing safety concerns	• Make plans for safety monitoring transparent to consumers
• Change record systems (e.g., integrate DMHI with the health record; integrate communication portal with tools practitioners use)	• Conduct small tests of the new processes
• Appropriate sufficient funds (e.g., to license the DMHI, initiate a contract, workflow integration, programming, staff training)	• Track time & resources spent implementing the DMHI
• Build partnerships for priority setting & evaluation	• Create learning collaboratives to share resources & learnings
Sustainment Phase	
• Optimize the technologies & implementation plans over time	• Assess changing needs & preferences over time

FIGURE 5-2 Implementation strategies for digital mental health
NOTE: DMHI refers to digital mental health intervention.
SOURCE: Reproduced from Graham et al., 2019. Copyright © 2019 by American Psychological Association. Reproduced with permission. Presented by Andrea Graham on June 9, 2022, at Accelerating the Use of Findings from Patient-Centered Outcomes Research in Clinical Practice to Improve Health and Health Care: A Workshop Series.

accounted for only 4 percent of the people who used the app and enrolled in the clinical trial. However, of those individuals who were referred to the app as the result of an EHR alert, 50 percent ended up participating in the clinical trial, compared to 4 percent of those reached via the direct-to-consumer approach. She noted this demonstrated the importance of the provider-patient interaction for digital tool uptake.

Graham said referral management is an important step in what she called the implementation cascade that first identifies people in need of care, convinces them to want the intervention, and then gets them to use it so they benefit from care (Graham et al., 2020c). One challenge to addressing this step is deciding who is responsible for integrating digital health tools into the workflow.

Graham concluded by highlighting important considerations for design of digital health tools. She said context and sustainability should be considered in the earliest phases of the design process. This includes considering how the implementation process for the digital tool will be integrated into clinical workflow. Developers should seek to allow end users to engage with new digital tools as soon as possible in the design process and evolve design in an iterative manner based on end user feedback.

DISCUSSION

Considerations for Assessing Digital Tools

Session moderator Cara Nikolajski, director of research design and implementation at the UPMC Center for High-Value Health Care, asked the panelists to discuss whether designers should assess apps in terms of evidence-based workflow integration, attention to equity, and other factors so that clinicians know which tools to prescribe over others. Krishnamurti replied that the Food and Drug Administration (FDA) does regulate digital apps that either diagnose or treat a health care issue. FDA also has the right to oversee and regulate other apps that do not fully meet that criterion. However, she noted that there are many tools available that have not gone through rigorous regulatory examination. She explained that was why her presentation highlighted some of the guiding principles as a framework for both designing and evaluating digital tools, as well as for the people who are evaluating whether they want to adopt a particular tool. Graham remarked on the importance of collaboration when thinking about how to engage with clinicians and how to ensure that they understand the tool and feel comfortable and confident referring patients to the tool. For example, her team has found that in certain primary care settings there is not much time to talk about mental health issues, nor are primary care providers comfortable doing so. This suggests there is a need to take a step back in training, engage with the clinical team, and talk about how to have those conversations.

Nikolajski then asked the group to discuss any standard metrics that the Agency for Health Research and Quality (AHRQ) should require for any implementation of a digital intervention. Schuster replied that in addition to outcomes, engagement rate should be evaluated. He noted the literature suggests that engagement rates with digital health tools are low unless accompanied by coaching or clinical service. Krishnamurti suggested a good engagement rate would likely depend on the function of the tool being evaluated. "If someone uses a tool sparsely but they get real value from it—maybe they log in once or twice in our tool, register intimate partner violence, and access support for that, that minimal use could have a big impact," she said. Krishnamurti said it is important to first define whom an app is designed to serve and how the app will serve them, and then develop the metric for engagement to capture who is using the tool and to what benefit. Schuster suggested a requirement to demonstrate a positive outcome at the population level, which will be contingent on engagement.

Opportunities to Combine Digital Tools and Community Health Workers

Another question from the audience asked the panelists to comment on possible opportunities for AHRQ to support combining digital tools with community health workers to provide care. Krishnamurti answered that digital tools represent an amazing opportunity to support community health workers and bridge gaps in health care. For example, digital tools might be useful for getting information from patients about risk factors that their physicians may not have the time to explore. They might also serve as a way in which community health workers can stay in touch with their clients and track their health issues. Krishnamurti said digital tools are complements to in-person care, not solutions on their own.

Graham agreed that digital tools are not a stand-alone solution. She noted that such tools can make it easier for clients to access more than one type of clinician, enhance health equity, and expand the diversity of whom the health care system can reach. It is important to be thoughtful about how data and opportunities to interact with a health care provider are integrated into the clinic workflow. "If patients are messaging all the time, who is responsible for reacting to that? Who is responsible for reading alerts and when in the workflow is it [message alert] going to pop up so that it can actually be really actionable?" she asked. She said that considering those factors is an important part of human-centered design, and they represent an important design implementation frontier the field needs to consider further.

Considering Equity when Designing Digital Tools

An audience member asked speakers to discuss strategies to address equity issues related to digital tools. Nikolajski noted both Graham and Krishnamurti discussed engaging stakeholders in the development process, which she said is one way to support advancing health equity. Schuster agreed and noted the need to ensure developers engage with communities that have health equity challenges and often access services less frequently than others. From an implementation science[2] perspective, said Graham, it is important to consider equity when creating and testing a tool that may not be equally available to all who might benefit from that tool. For example, researchers should consider the implications of providing a scale or cell phone to a study participant and then taking it back once the study is done. Krishnamurti pointed out that there are few opportunities to fund the dissemination and maintenance of digital tools. This is one reason, she said, why so many promising digital tools and decision support applications are built but not implemented.

CLOSING SUMMARY OF WORKSHOP 1

Lauren Hughes concluded the workshop by summarizing her takeaways from the presentations and discussions. She said several speakers highlighted several approaches for improving the design and implementation of research projects that are effective and generate trust and authenticity, intentionality, and longitudinal impact. Those include[3]

- co-creation with patients, families, and communities that are directly affected by a project;
- incorporating human-centered design approaches when designing interventions and involving a broad array of stakeholders and research colleagues; and
- including practice-based research networks (PBRNs) and community members as partners and respecting the expertise that community members bring to the research.

She said speakers also highlighted research and translation challenges that are important to identify and address to improve the impact of key research findings. These challenges include

---

[2] Implementation science is "the scientific study of methods to promote the systematic uptake of research findings and other EBPs [evidence-based practices] into routine practice, and, hence, to improve the quality and effectiveness of health services" (Bauer, 2015).

[3] These points were made by the individual workshop speakers/participants identified above. They are not intended to reflect a consensus among workshop participants.

- short funding cycles and funding sustainability;
- navigating complex adaptive systems that evolve during the course of research that can impact findings;
- developing effective approaches for disseminating research findings;
- increasing the use of effective digital tools that are designed for context, integrated smartly into workflows, and are engaging and valuable; and
- examining the design of studies to consider including mixed method approaches and more community-based participatory research.

She said another theme touched on by several speakers was the importance of continuing to challenge assumptions and consider new perspectives about engaging in patient-centered outcomes research (PCOR) and implementing PCOR findings. She highlighted several perspective related considerations for researchers that were put forth by speakers:[4]

- While facts are universal, implementation is local, so researchers should attend to local factors that will impact implementation.
- Community outreach begins with an answer, but community engagement ends with an answer.
- Privilege can contribute to psychological distortions, which can lead to an "us-versus-them" mentality that contributes to health inequities.
- Researchers should practice cultural humility and engage an assets-based rather than deficits-based approach when working and collaborating with communities.

---

[4] These points were made by the individual workshop speakers/participants identified above. They are not intended to reflect a consensus among workshop participants.

6

Workshop 2 Keynote: Community Engagement in PCOR for Health Equity

> **Key Messages Presented by Individual Speakers**
> - Cross-cutting strategies for achieving desired outcomes include training the next generation of researchers; building data, measurement, and analytic capacity; accelerating uptake of evidence in practice; and providing evidence to inform needed policy changes to sustain the implementation of interventions that produce outcomes that matter to patients and address health inequities. (Aguilar-Gaxiola)
> - Listening attentively to patient, family, and provider experiences is an important means of enhancing trust in the health care system. (Aguilar-Gaxiola)

INTRODUCTION

Lauren Hughes explained the second virtual workshop would start with a keynote presentation focusing on achieving equity through patient-centered outcomes research (PCOR) that includes meaningful community engagement. Subsequent sessions would discuss possibilities for collaborations among the Agency for Healthcare Research and Quality (AHRQ), the U.S. Department of Health and Human Services Assistant Secretary for Planning and Evaluation

(ASPE), and the Patient-Centered Outcomes Research Institute (PCORI) to improve health equity and the sustainability of their efforts.

Karin Rhodes, AHRQ, explained that AHRQ, ASPE, and PCORI worked independently in the first 10 years of the Patient-Centered Outcomes Research Trust Fund (PCORTF), but since Congress reauthorized PCORTF, the three agencies have begun collaborating more. AHRQ and PCORI, for example, created a joint workgroup to establish a common purpose, identify themes, develop strategic objectives, and prioritize opportunities to expand their collaborative efforts. One of AHRQ's strengths, she explained, is its infrastructure for reviewing and synthesizing evidence and translating that evidence to practice. AHRQ and PCORI have collaborated on dissemination and implementation projects as well as learning networks. She also described an example where an AHRQ evidence report identified new evidence gaps, so PCORI invested in research to address those gaps. The two agencies are also working together on training to address mutual priorities. Rhodes described a new AHRQ-PCORI scientist training program that is embedded in its learning health system. AHRQ and PCORI are targeting this training program at underserved communities, with an emphasis on primary care, by recruiting and training individuals from underrepresented and marginalized communities.

MEANINGFUL COMMUNITY ENGAGEMENT TO ADVANCE HEALTH EQUITY IN HEALTH SYSTEMS TRANSFORMATION

Sergio Aguilar-Gaxiola, professor of clinical internal medicine, founding director of the Center for Reducing Health Disparity, and director of the community engagement program at the University of California Davis Clinical Translational Science Center, noted that he is also co-chair of the National Academy of Medicine's (NAM's) organizing committee on Assessing Meaningful Community Engagement in Health and Health Care Programs and Policies. The goal of this project, said Aguilar-Gaxiola, was to consider how the committee might build effective, evidence-based, community-engaged indicators and metrics for measuring meaningful community engagement in a wide range of settings. Such indicators and metrics could then help shape how health care programs and policies are developed, implemented, and overseen, with special emphasis on those most in need. The organizing committee produced five resources: a conceptual model (released February 14, 2022), impact stories and videos, measurement instruments, a resource website,[1] and a NAM special publication that it will publish in fall 2022. Community engagement, the central feature of the conceptual model (Figure 6-1), emphasizes the criti-

---

[1] https://nam.edu/assessing-meaningful-community-engagement-a-conceptual-model-to-advance-health-equity-through-transformed-systems-for-health (accessed September 14, 2022).

cal importance of engaging and listening to communities and stakeholders to hear what matters to them regarding health, health care, and health equity. He noted that many of the same principles AHRQ includes in its strategic framework form the basis of the conceptual model. Trust, for example, appears throughout the model and its four domains: strengthened partnerships and alliances, expanded knowledge, thriving communities, and improved and sustainable health and health care programs. In addition to physical health, the model includes mental health, as well as community resilience and community power. Aguilar-Gaxiola said the central goal of the model is to achieve health equity through transformed systems for health by addressing the drivers of health; the drivers of change in health and health care; and the social, political, racial, economic, historical, and environmental context.

Aguilar-Gaxiola posed two questions for AHRQ to consider: How can AHRQ consider the elements of the National Academy of Medicine conceptual model for community engagement in its decision-making and strategic planning process structures as well as in the design and review of its funding opportunities for research dissemination and training? And, can AHRQ ask its funders, researchers, and institutions to consider this framework in project design?

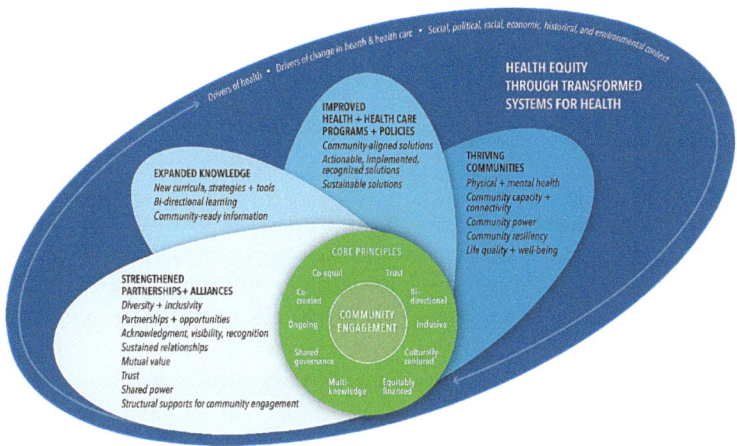

FIGURE 6-1 A conceptual model for assessing community engagement[a]

[a] See https://nam.edu/assessing-meaningful-community-engagement-a-conceptual-model-to-advance-health-equity-through-transformed-systems-for-health (accessed September 20, 2022).

SOURCE: Reproduced from the National Academies publication *Assessing Meaningful Community Engagement in Health & Health Care Programs & Policies* (2022). Presented by Sergio Aguilar-Gaxiola on June 17, 2022, at Accelerating the Use of Findings from Patient-Centered Outcomes Research in Clinical Practice to Improve Health and Health Care: A Workshop Series.

He then discussed several areas of alignment between the NAM model and AHRQ strategic framework. Those include goals related to

- Improving health equity,
- Improving patient and community engagement,
- Building trust and trustworthiness,
- Addressing mental health and the social determinants of health, and
- Promoting learning health systems and centers of excellence for development and advancement.

He added that the NAM conceptual model and the AHRQ strategic framework share several priorities, including

- training the next generation of researchers;
- building data, measurement, and analytic capacity;
- accelerating uptake of evidence in practice; and
- providing evidence to inform needed policy changes to sustain implementation of interventions that produce outcomes that matter to patients and address health inequities.

He closed by emphasizing the NAM model and its methods can support AHRQ's training of the next generation of patient-centered outcomes researchers.

DISCUSSION

Session moderator Jen Brown, cofounder and codirector of the Alliance for Research in Chicagoland Communities and lecturer in preventive medicine at Northwestern University, asked Aguilar-Gaxiola if he could further discuss how the community engagement model could help AHRQ develop its own community engagement mechanisms and structures that reflect elements of trustworthiness, co-creation, and shared power. He replied that the nation's experience during the COVID-19 pandemic pointed to the critical importance of trust and trustworthiness that has to be built through bidirectional relationships with various organizations and institutions by listening to and engaging the main stakeholders (the people being served) while considering their culture, language, and diversity. He noted that AHRQ's guiding principles include being patient centric, evidence based, collaborative, and stakeholder driven, as well as emphasizing continuous learning. Those principles, said Aguilar-Gaxiola, were central to the committee's assessment of meaningful community engagement.

Brown remarked that the commentary the committee released pointed out that the fundamental question is not whether entities think they are engaging communities, but whether communities feel engaged, which she noted is a powerful shift in perspective. She then asked Aguilar-Gaxiola to discuss how the committee operationalized that perspective in its work and if there were any lessons for AHRQ or this workshop. He replied that the steering committee that preceded the full organizing committee had a substantial change in perspective just by including—and listening to—community members, pointing to the importance of iterating based on community input.

An audience member asked Aguilar-Gaxiola to discuss how the community engagement conceptual model builds on community-oriented primary care (Institute of Medicine, 1983, 1984a, 1984b). He said there is alignment between the conceptual model and community-oriented primary care, both emphasize listening to patients and their families and building trust.

Brown noted that while it is important to work with a variety of stakeholders to have authentic, meaningful community engagement, that process can be complex, particularly when it comes to the power differential that can exist between stakeholders. She asked Aguilar-Gaxiola if he could discuss any lessons the model provides regarding this challenge while keeping with the principles of community engagement. He replied that the plurality and diversity of the stakeholders resemble a microcosm of what occurs in communities and even in families. The key, he said, is to be aware of those dynamics and communicate openly, authentically, and frankly to reach a common understanding of what matters for each particular stakeholder. In that regard, the NAM model and the guiding principles of community engagement can provide a roadmap for focusing on what matters and working toward system transformation that achieves health equity.

7

Workshop 2, Session 1: Possibilities for AHRQ–ASPE–PCORI Collaborations to Improve Health Equity

> **Key Messages Presented by Individual Speakers**
> - Reducing barriers for community based and patient advocacy organizations to access health care data should be part of efforts to improve health equity. (Puckrein)
> - Researchers should ensure data collected through community engagement is returned to that community in a form they find useful to improve community health. (Puckrein)
> - Opportunities for AHRQ to leverage PCORTF funding to advance health equity by supporting a research engagement infrastructure, prioritizing and requiring equity impact measurement in comparative effectiveness research, and building a pipeline of an equity-focused workforce through engagement. (Gaglioti)
> - Effective implementation requires considering how the research sample used for the evidence base matches or reflects the lived experiences of the populations and communities an intervention aims to help; the skill set and the capacity of the practitioners in real-world settings; and the dynamic and complex systems at the policy, community, and health systems level. (Shelton)
> - Reengineering the translation, dissemination, and implementation process for interventions requires that research, dissemination, implementation, and community partnership are all being done simultaneously in rapid dynamic cycles supported by data with a focus on outcomes and not just processes. (Rust)

Session moderator Brian Rivers, professor and director of the Cancer Health Equity Institute at Morehouse School of Medicine, explained presentations in this session would discuss approaches to create complementary collaborations among the Agency for Healthcare Research and Quality (AHRQ), the Office of the Assistant Secretary for Planning and Evaluation (ASPE), the Patient-Centered Outcomes Research Institute (PCORI), and other agencies to improve health equity. He noted that AHRQ's proposed strategic framework includes health equity as a high-priority component with desired outcomes that include reducing health disparities for AHRQ's priority populations, engaging underrepresented communities in training and implementation activities, and improving equity and access to needed care.

THE ROLE OF DATA IN HEALTH EQUITY

Gary Puckrein, founding president and chief executive officer of the National Minority Quality Forum (NMQF), explained that most of his organization's work centers on collecting health data and examining the intersection of policy and health outcomes. He explained that NMQF uses data to identify and address health inequity. He said limited access to health care data is a contributor to health inequity. He suggested AHRQ, ASPE, and PCORI could collaborate to democratize access to health care data as part of their efforts to address health inequity.

Puckrein said an important component of democratizing health care data is sharing data back with its creators so that they can manage their health appropriately. He noted that one access challenge is the sheer volume and complexity of health data, which creates difficulties for patient advocates seeking to access and use that data. This puts patient advocates at a disadvantage when they try to advocate for better health care and eliminate disparities. To address that challenge, his organization developed the patient advocacy learning community. This is an online geographic information system and data warehouse where his team is curating the data from 5 billion patient records and making it accessible to patient advocates in an easy-to-use format. The website also includes tools to analyze the data, with plans of augmenting them with artificial intelligence and other tools so that patient advocacy groups and community-based organizations can use the data to support their work. Puckrein closed by emphasizing health care is a data-driven system and everyone in the health care system needs to use data to get the best outcomes for patients.

STRENGTHENING THE PRIMARY CARE SYSTEM WHILE ADVANCING HEALTH EQUITY

Anne Gaglioti is associate professor of family medicine at Metro Health System and Case Western Reserve University's Population Health Research

Institute and associate professor at Morehouse School of Medicine's National Center for Primary Care (NCPC). She briefly described the framework that NCPC developed for applying a health equity lens to a learning health system approach for transforming health care organizations and communities. She said the foundational elements of the framework are to prioritize health equity, engage the community, target health disparities, act on the data, and learn and improve (Brooks et al., 2017).

Gaglioti also serves as co-director of the Southeast Regional Clinicians Network, an AHRQ practice-based research network (PBRN) of 203 federally qualified health centers serving over 4 million patients in eight southeastern U.S. states. She said PBRNs are well positioned to advance health equity because of the nature and structure of their operations, including their application of equity principles to their research. PBRNs engage patients, clinicians, and communities in their research. She explained PBRNs have an opportunity to measure the impact of programs and advance equity through their data, engagement, and dissemination infrastructure (Westfall et al., 2019).

Gaglioti offered suggestions for how AHRQ, ASPE, and PCORI might leverage Patient-Centered Outcomes Research Trust Fund (PCORTF) funding to advance health equity by supporting meaningful engagement with patients, clinicians, and communities. She noted these suggestions were informed by input from patient and stakeholder advisers. Her first suggestion was to support a research engagement infrastructure, given that engagement is foundational to equity. The Southeast Regional Clinician's Network has a high-level engagement infrastructure, but it is challenging to sustain because it depends on project funding. PCORTF funding could provide a mechanism for sustaining a longitudinal engagement infrastructure that would span projects and support building and sustaining trust and skills. This engagement infrastructure should incorporate capacity building for patient and stakeholder advisers and researchers, she said. She suggested that AHRQ should consider developing a space in which different stakeholder groups, patients, community members, community-based organization leaders, and clinician advisers could collaborate and have opportunities for shared learning and peer support.

Gaglioti's second suggestion was to prioritize and require equity impact measurement in comparative effectiveness research. She said applications for funding should ground their comparative effectiveness research and other implementation work in measuring disparities and evaluating the impact of the interventions on reducing disparities. She said this type of research should determine comparative effectiveness across different populations, and it should prioritize asking about comparative acceptability to different populations or the perceived sustainability or access to interventions for disproportionately impacted populations.

Her third suggestion was to build research and researcher capacity to support community engagement relationships that bolster trustworthiness. She suggested that career development awards should include a required or suggested training activity related to patient and stakeholder engagement in research. She added that PCORI's work around the science of engagement could inform and support that training. She also noted the importance of encouraging patient or community advisers with lived experience in the area of focus to serve as mentors on career development awards.

Gaglioti's fourth suggestion was to support engagement through the greater allocation of time as a resource. She explained engagement bolsters the opportunity for projects to cultivate equity. However, engagement requires a great deal of time to plan the work; align priorities; reach meaningful impact; and conduct, interpret, and disseminate the work. She suggested that grant applications should consider the time investment needed for effective engagement in their timelines. She explained that a longer timeline for developing an application on strong foundations of trust can be helpful, as would a long project period that supports more time for engagement across the spectrum of research processes.

Her final suggestion was to build the pipeline of an equity-focused workforce through engagement. She said the Jackson Heart Study does that well. When funding or designing a funding opportunity announcement focused on health equity, she suggested funding opportunities focused on health equity should require pipeline infrastructure focused on empowering youth or learners who are members of the disproportionately impacted group of interest. The pipeline infrastructure could consist of a mentorship program, scholar program, or internship.

Gaglioti closed by offering suggestions about equity-centered engagement in research and implementation from community partners involved in a project to mitigate the impact of COVID-19 on disproportionately impacted populations:

- Academic, private, and government partners should adapt their approaches based on input from community members in order to align their work with the needs of disproportionately affected communities.
- It is crucial that partnerships with community-based organizations are equitable with respect to meaningful leadership, agency, power, and funding support.
- Effort should be directed to sustain and build on the trust and partnerships across sectors that have developed during the COVID-19 pandemic so as not to squander this hard-earned, valuable trust.
- Include community representatives in the project governing board and leadership when planning and executing implementation projects designed for disproportionately affected populations.

ADDRESSING HEALTH EQUITY THROUGH DISSEMINATION AND IMPLEMENTATION SCIENCE

Rachel Shelton is associate professor of sociomedical sciences at Columbia University's Mailman School of Public Health and director of the implementation science initiative and co-director of the community engagement core resource at the Irving Institute for Clinical and Translational Research. She began by saying there is a well-documented, large gap between research and practice that has substantial implications for exacerbating social and health inequities. She noted that it can take 17 years for 14 percent of original research to impact patient care (Morris, 2011). Shelton opined this is in part because the research community often takes a passive approach to dissemination.

Shelton said the inconsistent uptake of COVID-19 vaccination in the United States has demonstrated evidence alone does not lead to widespread or equitable uptake or adoption. Research evidence is only one component to consider when planning uptake and implementation at scale. She said effective and equitable dissemination and implementation requires the following:

- considering how the evidence base matches or reflects the lived experiences of the populations and communities an intervention aims to help;
- the skill set and the capacity of the practitioners beyond the research setting; and
- the dynamic and complex systems at the policy, community, and health systems level (Brownson et al., 2009; Green et al., 2009).

Shelton explained dissemination and implementation science seeks to translate research and evidence into policy and practice with the goal of impacting population health equitably and at scale. It involves the scientific study of methods, strategies, and frameworks to better assess context and actively promote routine adoption, use, and sustainability of evidence-based interventions and practices in real-world clinical, community, and public health settings to improve the quality of care and health (Eccles and Mittman, 2006). She noted that there is a distinction between dissemination and implementation. Dissemination refers to how to deliver evidence and evidence-based programs to key stakeholders, leadership, and decision makers. Implementation refers to how to integrate and deliver evidence and evidence-based programs in diverse, real-world settings and provide the capacity to deliver those interventions at scale. Shelton explained that implementation typically occurs at the end of the traditional research process after generating the evidence base. That evidence base is frequently developed in academic settings that may not reflect the experience of significant structural barriers and structural inequities that contribute to health inequity. She said addressing the disconnect between the evidence base and implementation efforts requires thinking early in the research process about creating that evidence base with a focus on community engagement and equity.

Shelton said equity-oriented implementation requires paying explicit attention to culture, context, history, values, assets, and the strengths of the community and ensuring those are integrated into the foundation of how research is conducted. She explained equity-oriented implementation requires prioritizing and building an evidence base that explicitly addresses health inequities, promotes equity, and addresses the root and structural causes of those inequities (Baumann and Cabassa, 2020; Baumann and Long, 2021). Achieving an equity orientation requires investing in the development and implementation of evidence-based interventions that build capacity among patient systems and communities and actively seek to promote health equity. She said equity-oriented implementation also requires reflecting on the evidence base and asking the following questions:

- Has the intervention been found to be effective among a population and setting experiencing inequities?
- Does the intervention reflect the lived experiences of communities impacted by structural inequities?
- How can the intervention be culturally adapted or contextually adapted?
- Is the intervention effective at reducing health inequities and promoting health equity?
- Does the intervention build community capacity?
- Does the intervention address social or structural determinants, such as discrimination, stigma, mistrust, and racism?
- Does the intervention work across sectors to address multilevel upstream policy, systems, and community levels?

Shelton said equity-oriented implementation requires changing the notion of what counts as an evidence-based intervention to incorporate consideration of who is involved in the development of that evidence base, and engaging communities and patients at the beginning to address issues of feasibility and acceptability (Bailey et al., 2017; Brownson et al., 2022; Mazzucca et al., 2021). She added that this requires considering both the scientific hierarchy of evidence as well as practice-based evidence and learning from community settings such as schools and faith-based organizations. She explained that grounding an intervention in the community enhances the focus on issues of flexibility, cost, relevance, and accounting for the local social and cultural context. This approach also helps the process reflect local strengths and solutions and enhance benefits to the community. She described an example of her experience partnering with a group of Black lay health advisers and cancer survivors. She noted how important it has been to understand that, at least in part, they mistrusted the changing guidelines around breast and cervical cancer screening because the clinical trials that have informed many of the guidelines have not reflected their lived experience of having more aggressive tumors at younger ages (Shelton et al., 2021).

Shelton suggested funding organizations could support opportunities for researchers to consider adaptations that support health equity when they are building an evidence base. She said when building an evidence base, researchers should consider how they adapt programs to address some of the social determinants of health by adjusting where they are delivered, who delivers them, and how they support or enhance issues of health equity. She suggested funding organizations could also prioritize developing and testing dissemination and implementation strategies that build capacity and reach settings and populations equitably. She highlighted a need to build an evidence base for how to facilitate widespread and equitable dissemination. She said that building that evidence base requires identifying key adopters, stakeholders, and trusted messengers and their key characteristics across diverse settings. It also requires understanding the characteristics that influence the speed and extent of adoption (Kwan et al., 2022a; Stewart et al., 2018). She posited that health equity training could be included in implementation to reduce bias and promote health equity in health care systems.

Shelton said enhancing equity requires focusing on reach and representation from the beginning of the implementation process (Baumann et al., 2011). She said context matters when developing an implementation strategy, noting bias that exists within the clinical algorithms embedded in health systems. She suggested researchers and funders should be accountable for ensuring that research reflects a wide range of settings, populations, and providers, because that will shape the nature of the evidence base. She said community partners should be included in the process of developing metrics related to measuring an implementation project's impact on health equity. She added that when planning implementation researchers should consider what will be meaningful, valuable, and important to the community; and how to return data to the community in a form that is accessible and actionable (Baumann and Cabassa, 2020; Proctor et al., 2011).

Shelton explained she has used the Reach, Effectiveness, Adoption, Implementation, and Maintenance (RE-AIM) evaluation and planning framework to bring an equity lens to considerations about who is reached, which settings are reached, and which populations and settings are able to implement and maintain an intervention. The RE-AIM framework has also helped her be transparent throughout her work so as to be accountable when and where inequities arise (Shelton et al., 2020).

As a final comment, she encouraged everyone to think about how to accelerate the progress toward health equity and advance equitable impact at scale. She said doing so will require collaborating, investing, and advancing both meaningful community engagement and implementation science.

COMMUNITY PARTNERSHIPS IN RESEARCH

George Rust is professor of behavioral sciences and social medicine and director of the Florida State University College of Medicine's Center for Medicine and Public Health and medical executive director for the Lyonne County Health Department. He began by noting that in the 7 years since he worked at AHRQ, there has been a beneficial shift in health care research beyond a focus on patients in the health care setting to considering whole people in a community context; moving from looking at one disease at a time to all forms of complexity, and from disparities to equity. He also appreciates increased engagement in multidimensional interventions in health care research, and that scientific methodology now includes dynamic interventions that change during the course of a research project. He also suggested AHRQ should consider furthering these efforts through developing a center for primary care research. He also suggested primary care related research could benefit from explicit funding for the National Center of Excellence on Primary Care, as well as regional centers for primary care research around the country.

Rust recounted that he began his career working at a migrant community health center funded by a program the Office of Economic Opportunity program started in the 1960s. That program sent funds directly to community organizations, which shifted the power dynamics toward the community. He suggested agencies funding health care research should consider a similar approach. Rust opined, "I think we need to think about models and mechanisms in which we can make that happen, so that it is not at the university level or investigator-initiated level to decide how much power sharing is going to happen or engaged the community is going to be. Real partners share the money, real partners share the power, real partners share control." He encouraged workshop participants to move away from framing a challenge encountered when attempting to engage with a community as one of community trust, instead framing it as a matter of researchers' trustworthiness. He emphasized that addressing power dynamics between researchers and communities need to be addressed before trustworthiness can be addressed. Rust referred the workshop participants to the American Association of Medical College's principles of trustworthiness for additional information.

Rust called for reengineering the notion that translation, dissemination, and implementation is a linear process. He proposed an approach in which research, dissemination, implementation, and community partnership are all being done simultaneously in rapid dynamic cycles. He said if done with a focus on outcomes and not just processes, this new approach would result in dissemination and implementation happening at the same time as the research, supporting an iterative process. Rust stressed the importance of data supporting plan-do-study-act (PDSA) cycles and changing research interventions rapidly in response to feedback. This requires data to support rapid feedback loops that include repeated measures of actionable information at the local level. These measures will provide granular demographic and clinical strata. He added additional work is needed to develop vertically proportionate diversity among research agencies, universities and other institutions, and investigators.

Rust described Morehouse School of Medicine's Prevention Research Center as an example of an effective approach to building a community partnership. He noted that Morehouse School of Medicine's Prevention Research Center spent a year working with the community, not to develop its principles of community engagement but for the community to develop its principles of university engagement (Box 7-1). Rust closed by suggesting researchers should benchmark progress against an ultimate outcome of optimal and equitable health for all with an affirmative expectation that a project must achieve equity.

BOX 7-1
One Community's Guiding Principles for University Engagement

1. Policies and programs should be based on mutual respect and justice for all people, free from discrimination or bias.
2. All people have a right to political, economic, cultural, and environmental self-determination.
3. The community has the right to participate as an equal partner at every level of decision-making including needs assessment, planning, implementation, enforcement, and evaluation.
4. Principles of individual and community informed consent should be strictly enforced.
5. The community repudiates the targeting of people of color and lower socioeconomic status for the purpose of testing reproductive and medical procedures and vaccinations.

continued

> **BOX 7-1 CONTINUED**
>
> 6. Present and future generations should be provided an education that emphasizes social and environmental issues, based on our experience and an appreciation of our diverse cultural perspectives.
> 7. Research processes and outcomes should benefit the community. Community members should be hired and trained whenever possible and appropriate, and the research should help build and enhance community assets.
> 8. Community members should be a part of the analysis and interpretation of data and should have input into how the results are distributed.
> 9. Productive partnerships between researchers and community members should be encouraged to last beyond the life of the project. This will make it more likely that research findings will be incorporated into ongoing community programs and therefore provide the greatest possible benefit to the community from research.
> 10. Community members should be empowered to initiate their own research projects, which address needs they identify themselves.
>
> SOURCE: Presented by George Rust on June 17, 2022 at Accelerating the Use of Findings from Patient-Centered Outcomes Research in Clinical Practice to Improve Health and Health Care: A Workshop Series (Morehouse School of Medicine, 2022).

DISCUSSION

Community Partnerships and Engagement

Rivers asked the group to discuss strategies for better understanding and ensuring community responsiveness in implementation and dissemination work. Shelton said one important component of that strategy is long-term and flexible funding. She added that researchers should be explicit about their long-term goals, expect their research to address community priorities, and identify how that research relates to health equity. She suggested the above should be included as part of funding announcements and review criteria. She also suggested considering funding for project-agnostic infrastructure that supports engagement and continuity of relationships over time.

An audience member noted that the National Academy of Medicine recently shared a commentary about the need for community empowerment and asked the speakers to discuss how researchers and funders could support community empowerment more effectively (Farhang and Morales, 2022). Rust replied that HRSA and its federally qualified health centers provide a good model for putting power in the hands of community-owned organizations. He said HRSA has developed strategies that set boundaries, that ensure funds are spent appropriately and tracked correctly; and ensure professional standards are met while empowering consumer-majority boards.

Gaglioti added that one of the most important approaches to support community empowerment is to align projects with priorities identified by patient and stakeholder advisory boards. She also suggested that medical and graduate schools should offer courses in academic humility.[1] She opined that research grants are often not structured well for sharing power or resources. She suggested incorporating longer-term funding mechanisms that state explicitly that community partners are not just investigators but can be co-leaders, which should facilitate access to resources.

Rivers asked Puckrein how community empowerment could help generate data that is patient or community facing and responsive to the needs of different communities. Puckrein said one structural problem is patient advocacy groups do not have the capacity to go through the audit required when receiving a federal grant exceeding $750,000. He suggested funding agencies will need to address that barrier to improve access to funds for community-based organizations. In terms of data to meet community needs, Puckrein would like to build what he referred to as a community data lake that would give communities access to the data and the analytical capabilities to make use of the data. He said the success of an intervention that a community chooses to implement depends on having good data. Academic institutions can play a role by helping communities manage the data and turn it into useful information.

Rivers thanked Rust for being explicit about calling out issues of power and acknowledging the roles researchers play in actuating that problem. He asked Rust how he envisions the role of government agencies to solve this issue and address equity. Rust replied that power sharing requires restructuring the grant funding process, including the grant review and peer-review processes at the university level. Rust said accountability is imperative for eliminating outcome disparities, and researchers need to have flexibility to engage in rapid cycle change with an affirmative expectation of moving forward.

---

[1] Also referred to as Intellectual Humility, academic and intellectual humility is defined as (a) having insights about the limits of one's knowledge, marked by an openness to alternative ideas, and (b) the ability to present one's ideas non-offensively and receive information non-defensively (Wong and Wong, 2021).

Primary Care Research Planning

Rivers noted that the National Center for Excellence in Primary Care Research received $2 million in funding in 2022 and the President's budget calls for $10 million, but less than 1 percent of federal research funding goes to primary care, and he asked Rust how a PCOR partnership could improve funding for primary care research. Rust replied that current funding, even though small, is a good start as it represents an acknowledgment of the importance of primary care research. He said it also provides a foundation on which to build. Rust suggested that researchers should build on that foundation by beginning to develop plans for effective use of future funding, including the connections and research centers to build, and the research networks closest to the front lines that are most likely to be doing research that will be implemented as it is being done.

Possibilities for Collaborations for Health Equity

Concluding the discussion, Rivers asked each panelist to briefly summarize their ideas for possibilities for collaboration among AHRQ, ASPE, and PCORI to improve and create new models that advance health equity. Shelton said it will be important to have a clear, synergistic, and explicit definition of what health equity means, since it means different things to different groups. That definition can then translate into expectations for grant funding, metrics, and prioritizing evidence-based interventions. Gaglioti encouraged the agencies to use their longitudinal funding to support infrastructure for project-agnostic engagement and partnership infrastructure that prioritizes equity in the measurement of comparative effectiveness research, builds researcher capacity around how to partner and engage, and gives time for those relationships to develop. She also suggested funding infrastructure to build a pipeline of people in the community who can engage in the work of advancing health equity. Puckrein suggested the agencies provide more resources to meet underserved community needs and to build a data infrastructure to support the work that will take place in those communities. Rust suggested each agency should ensure it operationalizes its core values in all of its grant funding mechanisms and review processes.

8

Workshop 2, Session 2: Opportunities for AHRQ, ASPE, PCORI Collaborations to Improve Sustainability of Their Efforts

> **Key Messages Presented by Individual Speakers**
> - Technical support and building relationships are important factors for successful community-based data collection systems. (Collier)
> - Strategic thinking about research objectives, questions, data collection, and resources can help AHRQ better align with state policy makers' needs. (Blewett)
> - Research is needed to develop measures and mechanisms to capture valid and reliable self-report data of race and ethnicity, sexual orientation and gender identity, and disability status that can be incorporated into PCOR. (Blewett)
> - The setting in which data is collected must be considered before it is incorporated into a clinical decision support model for care in a different setting. Data is not always applicable across settings. (Phillips)

MAINTAINING PARTNERSHIPS FOR SUSTAINABLE DATA COLLECTION

Abby Collier, director of the National Center for Fatality Review and Prevention, explained that her organization, a program of the Michigan Public Health Institute, supports all aspects of child fatality review, as well as of fetal and infant mortality review.[1] These reviews are community-based processes that seek to understand the circumstances of a child fatality. This work supports state and local programs in terms of training, technical assistance, and written guidance. They also maintain a national data system. The center is tasked with building continuity between and within these programs across the United States. It also provides a connected data network for more than 1,500 U.S. fatality review teams and provides linkages to national and state resources to help teams translate their findings into action.

One unique role the center plays is collecting real-time, community-based data by reviewing individual fatalities. When the team gathers to review individual cases, each team member shares what they know about the child, family, and community that is relevant to the death. After completing the review process, the team enters the data into their national database. Both this data as well as the content of their qualitative discussions are used to write recommendations for prevention at the local, state, and national levels. Collier noted that there is a great deal of variability in child death review. Some states have a comprehensive process. However, other states have an inconsistent approach in which not all communities conduct a comprehensive review. There are approximately 2,700 users across the United States, making data consistency and quality a challenge. States have varying resources for collecting and entering data and their child death review committees have varying access to records. Collier explained that currently 47 states use the center for child death reviews, and 18 of those use it for child death reviews and fetal and infant mortality reviews. She explained that child death review creates an opportunity to look at these sentinel events though a systems-level lens, which can be beneficial to the local community. She noted that child death reviews are not intended to place blame, but rather to look for opportunities to improve how systems work.

The success of the data system, said Collier, depends on relationships. The center prioritizes functionality for end users when making decisions related to the case reporting system. They also work to promote flexibility and ease of access for use; states, for example, are able to add individual questions to their inputs. Center staff assist users in reducing data entry burden by collaborating to prioritize the data they collect and enter. Center staff also review data quality and provide feedback to the users. Finally, the center created a data dashboard to empower state-level review teams that do not have extensive epidemiology skills or resources. The center also uses feedback from state teams to determine the focus of their national reports.

She noted that problem solving and technical support has helped the center build trust with the state-level child death review teams. Those efforts

---

[1] Details available at https://ncfrp.org (accessed September 14, 2022).

have also allowed the center to learn strategies that can be applied in other states facing similar challenges.

STATE-LEVEL DATA COLLABORATIONS

Lynn Blewett, professor in the School of Public Health and director of the State Health Access Data Assistance Center (SHADAC) at the University of Minnesota, began her presentation by explaining that from a state-level health policy perspective, the promotion of health equity requires a different approach than traditional clinical effectiveness research. This is because states have different objectives, different research questions, and different data resources. The goal of her presentation, then, was to encourage the Agency for Healthcare Research and Quality (AHRQ) to think strategically about how to influence and engage with state policy makers.

Blewett said that in many states, health policy focuses on equity, access, affordability of care and how to better engage priority populations to improve population health. State health policy also strives to incentivize health plans to facilitate high-quality care to people with low incomes via Medicaid, as well as identify the factors that impede access to affordable, equitable care. Policy can be developed based on the policy levers available. These include

- Medicaid eligibility and payment policy,
- managed care organization contract requirements,
- regulating the private commercial health insurance market,
- financing the state employee health plans,
- financing, and
- state cost growth benchmarking and other cost-control strategies.

She encouraged AHRQ to take its focus on equity seriously and to think strategically about how to use its resources to address equity challenges. Targeting equity requires measuring and understanding who these people are and including them in state data resources. She encouraged AHRQ, the Office of the Assistant Secretary for Planning and Evaluation (ASPE), and the Patient-Centered Outcomes Research Institute (PCORI) to focus their investments on supporting projects on these populations, include an equity lens, and consider data development and infrastructure for state Medicaid data and public programs.

Blewett emphasized the need for reliable, self-reported data on race and ethnicity. Self-reported data on race and ethnicity can be a powerful tool for Medicaid programs to measure social determinants of health and address health equity. However, research on how to collect such data is nascent, and collecting that data is challenging for providers and insurers. ASPE has completed some work on imputation of race and ethnicity, but states are reluctant to use such methods because of concerns about transparency and difficulty engaging communities about the methodology (Branham et al., 2022). She suggested that Patient-Centered Outcomes Research Trust Fund (PCORTF) investments could support further development of measures to fill gaps in existing Medicaid claims data, electronic health record (EHR) data, and other claims-based data resources. SHADAC is working with state Medicaid data analysts on a project investigating how best to encourage Medicaid beneficiaries to share what are currently optional data on race, ethnicity, sexual orientation, gender identity, and disability status. They hope to translate those findings into best practices and policy change. Key components of engaging with Medicaid beneficiaries in that project included building trust and explaining what purpose the data will serve in terms of identifying and addressing health disparities. Blewett emphasized the need for additional funding for research on best practices and translating research into policy. She also would like to see the U.S. Office of Management and Budget (OMB) expand its efforts on the development of standards for race and ethnicity data, provide guidance to the states on flexibility, and provide incentives for state engagement in efforts to collect more granular and disaggregated data. She said that in 2019 the Centers for Medicare and Medicaid Services (CMS) released the Transformed Medicaid Statistical Information System (T-MSIS), which reports CMS-collected state Medicaid data. While quality is improving with these data there are still areas of concern about completeness in some critical areas. For example, 30 states did not submit acceptable data for inpatient managed care encounters, and 22 states submitted race and ethnicity data whose quality was of high concern or unusable. Additionally, access to the system is expensive. Blewett said there is a continued need to support state data capacity and provide incentives to collect better quality data. She noted that data would provide important insights on social determinants of health not typically found in EHRs or medical claims data.

Blewett highlighted another project, the Medicaid Outcomes Distributed Research Network (MODRN), which involves a group of states working together on a distributed research protocol (Adams et al., 2019; Zivin et al., 2022). Participating states work together on programming, conduct their own analysis on their data, and then submit tables with deidentified data to investigators at the University of Pittsburgh, who conduct further analysis. This approach avoids the need for data privacy and data use agreements because the states do the necessary programming with their own data. The MODRN team has used these data in projects on opioid use disorder that led to recommendations for Medicaid reforms (Donohue et al., 2022; Jarlenski et al., 2021; Kennedy and Sheets, 2021; Medicaid Outcomes Distributed Research Network, 2021).

Blewett described the Massachusetts Medicaid program which adjusts payments to health plans based on barriers to economic, food, and housing security using a hybrid approach that combines administrative data and American Community Survey data. This social risk-adjustment method uses an index developed with variables from the survey. It includes enrollees' addresses to develop census block indicators, a neighborhood stress score, and a measure of housing instability based on International Classification of Diseases (ICD) social determinants of health Z codes for housing insecurity. An early evaluation of this program found that including social determinants and related variables with risk scores strengthens the predictive power of risk adjustment and yields more accurate payments to managed care organizations (Jones and Muller, 2018). She said these results suggest that states may be able to encourage the use of Z codes by requiring managed care organizations to enter into value-based care arrangements with providers and by clarifying the rules governing providers' collection and use of social needs data.

Blewett noted that it would be beneficial for AHRQ to support research on the role of community context, poverty, structural racism, and the social determinants of health in health outcomes. She noted there is also limited understanding of the complex network of safety-net providers that are often unrepresented in clinical trials or comparative effectiveness research. These providers serve patients from groups that have historically been made vulnerable and other priority populations and provide unique access to needed care. Another opportunity for research is investigating the role of Medicaid strategies in increasing access to quality care for its enrolled populations.

She concluded her presentation with a list of possible priorities for AHRQ research funding, which included the following:

- Patient-centered outcomes research (PCOR) studies to examine the intersection of the social determinants of health and clinical health indicators to gain greater understanding of their impact on disease burden.
- Projects that develop partnerships between state or local data organizations and local researchers, such as the State University Partnership Learning Network and MODRN, to answer relevant policy questions and build data infrastructure.
- Projects that develop regional social needs indexes.
- Promote collaboration between state policy organizations that engage with community stakeholders and policy makers to set research priorities and find opportunities for evaluation research to inform policy making.
- Research that includes the development of measures and mechanisms to capture valid and reliable self-reported data of race, ethnicity, sexual orientation, gender identity, and disability status.

AHRQ–ASPE–PCORI COLLABORATIONS TO IMPROVE EFFORT SUSTAINABILITY

Robert Phillips Jr., executive director of the Center for Professionalism and Value in Health Care at the American Board of Family Medicine, discussed examples of future opportunities for collaboration among AHRQ, ASPE, and PCORI with an emphasis on sustainable projects. The first is a collaboration among the American Board of Family Medicine, Stanford University, and the U.S. Census Bureau to develop a "gold standard" small area deprivation index, analogous to the neighborhood stress score that Massachusetts Medicaid uses as part of its risk-adjustment process. These indexes would be predictive for clinical quality, costs and use, prevalence of health conditions, and mortality at the census block group level. Researchers would compare existing deprivation indexes to understand their usefulness for payment policy and for clinical application in public health. The project aims to create a research bench, using data from the Federal Statistical Research Data Centers. One of the benefits of a research bench is that it has secure access and authorization controls. It would also enable harnessing the analytic capacity of external partners such as universities that is not available inside the U. S. Department of Health and Human Services (HHS). The current project plans for the Census Bureau to become the data steward that maintains this resource. The current project builds on an ASPE–AHRQ collaboration on county-level social determinants of health data. Phillips then posed three questions regarding this project:

1. What if PCORTF dollars brought identified data sets together in these research data centers to create a bench of resources so that questions could be answered rapidly?
2. What if federal data strategy authority allowed a core of key health data assets to be maintained for authorized access and those assets did not require 12 to 18 months to assemble?
3. What if a "lab bench" of HHS data assets were available to authorized users to answer the nation's most pressing health equity questions and to create new tools for policy use?

The second collaboration Phillips discussed would create a "wet lab" for artificial intelligence and machine learning (AI/ML) that would focus on analyzing primary care data. He explained that more than half of all outpatient visits occur in the primary care setting. However, a large majority of data that researchers use to develop AI/ML-based clinical decision support tools does not come from the primary care setting, which lacks capacity to support such projects. Phillips contended that applying decision support tools developed using hospital data to decision-making in primary care could harm people. In contrast, the wet lab would use data from primary care to develop and test clinical decision support tools. Those tools would then need to meet a certification requirement prior to incorporation into an EHR. He added that this project is consistent with the goals and priorities of AHRQ, ASPE, and PCORI. This project has the potential to generate an AI/ML-powered tool that would calibrate a new clinical decision support tool using data in a health system's EHR.

The American Board of Family Medicine Foundation has allocated $3 million for three projects to build needed capacity:

1. A 5-year effort to increase capacity in family medicine departments.
2. Exploratory efforts to link doctoral students or postdoctoral scholars who have expertise in AI/ML to work one-on-one with primary care researchers.
3. Ongoing support for infrastructure development for an AI/ML learning collaborative at Stanford University's Center for Population Health Studies.

Phillips noted that the Gordon and Betty Moore Foundation has expressed interest in joining this effort. He suggested that expanding this collaboration is an opportunity for PCORTF.

Another collaboration focuses on outcomes from federal investments in the clinician workforce. Currently, only $500 million of the $19 billion that Medicare, Medicaid, and the Veterans Health Administration (VHA) spend annually on clinician training requires outcome assessments. The size of the primary care workforce is decreasing, particularly in rural areas and in outpatient settings (Phillips et al., 2022). He said that a recent study linked a 1-year decrease in life expectancy for people living in rural areas with health professional shortages in the rural primary care workforce. Another study released in May 2022 found that only 10 percent of people trained in internal medicine are going into outpatient primary care. He posited that AHRQ, ASPE, and PCORI could collaborate to support efforts to investigate and address the primary care workforce shortage.

The final collaboration Phillips addressed would update, reconfigure, and revive clinical data infrastructure. In 2018, the National Ambulatory Medical Care Survey (NAMCS) initially included 2,999 physicians, but lost 1,352 of them to follow-up because they did not meet the inclusion criteria. The response rate of the remaining 1,647 eligible physicians was approximately 40 percent. Phillips noted that led to a small sample size on which to base the survey findings.[2] The Centers for Disease Control and Prevention (CDC) con-

---

[2] Full demographics can be found at https://www.cdc.gov/nchs/data/ahcd/namcs_summary/2018-namcs-web-tables-508.pdf (accessed September 14, 2022).

vened an NAMCS workgroup in 2021 that recommended evolving NAMCS to include a broader diversity of ambulatory care providers to more completely capture what is happening in ambulatory care. The workgroup also recommended looking for other opportunities to create longitudinal sampling. Phillips suggested that AHRQ, ASPE, and PCORI consider how they could collaborate to support efforts to improve NAMCS and supplement it with registry data, claims data, and EHR data to create a more valuable data set that is more representative of the care provided in the primary care setting.

Phillips acknowledged Puckrein's comments about data infrastructure and creating a data lake and noted that there has been a significant loss of community health indicators as a result of the end of four federal health data systems in 2016. One such tool, the Community Health Status Indicators tool, was a reliable source of standardized, local health data for communities during its two decades of operation. Many stakeholders have called for a replacement tool that would enable local health needs assessments, peer comparisons, and the capacity to create communities of solutions locally (Phillips et al., 2021). Phillips wondered how PCORTF investments could support such an effort and if it could be a product of the collaboration between the Census Bureau and the Federal Statistical Research Data Centers that he discussed at the start of his presentation.

DISCUSSION

Supporting Data Stewardship, Access, and Quality

Session moderator Megan Daugherty Douglas, assistant professor of community health and preventive medicine at the Morehouse School of Medicine and director of research and policy at the Morehouse School of Medicine's National Center for Primary Care, asked Blewett to discuss the role that SHADAC and other data infrastructures can play in data stewardship and improving or supporting improvement in the timeliness, access, and quality of the data. Blewett replied that she has seen some progress in the federal government related to obtaining more accurate race and ethnicity data and to provide more guidance on standards and methods to acquire better self-reported data. She added that states are using the data that they can access, including the administrative data from their public programs, to inform immediate policy decisions. She explained that states submit their data to T-MSIS, then use another, more granular data set to conduct their own analysis, which may or may not replicate what they send to the federal government. Blewett would focus initial efforts on determining how to best incentivize states to collect race and ethnicity data and on helping providers understand how best to encourage people to provide self-reported race and ethnicity data.

Douglas asked Collier to discuss the importance of the collaborations and relationships that go into data reporting, quality, and timeliness and how to think about scaling those best practices. Collier explained that collaborations and relationships are critical to quality and timely data reporting. She noted that good relationships make it possible for her organization to work with its partners to address conflicting or missing data; while legislation around information sharing exists, it cannot force agencies to provide quality data.

Phillips said that when he served on the National Committee on Vital and Health Statistics, there were discussions about what is needed improve the quality of data submitted to these data sets. One clear message from stakeholders was the need to show them how their data would be used. He added that collaborations and relationships are critical for ensuring that these data sets support interventions and activities that matter in the communities providing the data.

A question from the audience asked the panelists to discuss their ideas for collaboration between AHRQ, ASPE, and PCORI to address the need for improved quality of data collected in EHRs, as well as challenges in moving information across the health care system using health information exchanges. Blewett said that the nation's multipayer system has added complexity to combining data across systems. As a result, real time data from health information exchanges would be difficult to implement. She noted that Minnesota does not have a functional health information exchange because many of the state's health systems use the Epic EHR, which can be used to share data between health systems already. Her team has worked with a state-level all-payer claims database that has some capacity to do cross-payer analysis with Medicare, Medicaid, and the commercial market. However, that database is missing data from self-insured plans.

Phillips commented that health information exchanges were well-envisioned but have challenges around execution, limited participation, and sustainability efforts. He noted that the all-claims payer databases could be a good resource. He suggested that these databases could represent another opportunity for AHRQ, ASPE, and PCORI to collaborate on projects to support data infrastructure and application.

Considering End Users of Health Care Data

Douglas then asked the speakers to explain who they see as the end users of health care data. Phillips explained that the examples that he discussed focused on clinicians and policy makers as end users. He noted that policy makers can use this data to adjust Medicaid managed care payments so that more resources flow to patients and clinicians in systematically divested communities. He added that clinicians seek to use data to improve the quality of the care they provide. Blewett noted that researchers and Medicaid agency representatives were interested in using data from the Medicaid equity dashboard project. She added that Medicaid staff are interested in using data to compare their work with that in other states and to learn from one another.

Douglas asked Collier to discuss how the National Center for Fatality Review and Prevention assesses different users' ability to use and analyze the data themselves versus relying on the support that the center provides. Collier replied that the center offers new users the opportunity to meet with staff. This gives center staff an opportunity to ascertain the degree of support the new user will need. In addition, center staff engages its network to obtain feedback about user needs and opportunities to improve the reporting system.

Elaborating on the AI/ML Wet Lab

Phillips was asked to elaborate on the AI/ML wet lab he described in his presentation. He provided an example of a possible use for the wet lab. Currently, most research into long COVID uses data from hospital or subspecialty clinic EHRs. As a result, all of that data are coming from people who are already diagnosed with long COVID when they arrive in those settings. That approach does not include data from the primary care setting where patients initially present with undifferentiated symptoms and without a long COVID diagnosis. He noted that patients with long COVID present to primary care with a variety of symptoms that clinicians must differentiate from symptoms of heart or lung disease. The data captured during that process in primary care could be used in AI/ML to develop clinical decision support tools informed by more longitudinal data.

Considerations for Expanding Use of Z Codes

Douglas next asked what is needed to expand the use of Z codes. Phillips replied that payment policy would be an effective method to increase use. He added that reimbursement for using Z codes is an important incentive, but a more important reason to use Z codes is that they can help clinicians better identify and address the barriers related to the social determinants of health experienced by their patients. He suggested that integrating this information into EHRs could increase the likelihood of a clinician asking a patient about barriers related to the social determinants of health they may be experiencing. The addition of this information in EHRs to a payment policy that incentivized use of Z codes could increase their use.

He noted that Massachusetts is conducting a demonstration project to test that hypothesis. Massachusetts has established a funding model in which clinicians that identify patients experiencing barriers related to the social determinants of health can refer that patient to community-based organizations (CBOs) for relevant support. The funds follow the patient, meaning that in this funding model, instead of the clinician receiving reimbursement, the CBOs are reimbursed based on the support they provide to each patient. The Community Care Cooperative, the managed care organization of 18 federally qualified health centers in Massachusetts, has developed a data platform that manages the identification, referral, and feedback loop for people receiving support through this model. The cooperative covers 12.5 percent of all patients in the state who are eligible based on the neighborhood stress score. Providers in the cooperative account for 80 percent of the referrals in the model, primarily because they have an infrastructure to identify and track those individuals. Phillips suggested that this could be an opportunity for AHRQ to support research to identify the data infrastructure needed to disseminate this type of program widely. Blewett agreed with this idea and said it could help address health equity in AHRQ's priority populations.

Speakers' Final Thoughts

Douglas then asked the panelists to share their final thoughts. Blewett replied that AHRQ could benefit from engaging state level policy makers and analysts to learn from their work related to the social determinants of health and the effect of structural racism on health equity. Phillips highlighted the opportunity that AHRQ has for helping turn data into information and tools for communities and policy makers. Collier reiterated that child death review teams are an opportunity to see how systems work when they are tested and an opportunity to make profound community change in a fairly real-time format. She emphasized that engaging with child death review from a data perspective is important, but it is also an opportunity to learn how different systems can effectively collaborate, particularly when they are under pressure.

CLOSING SUMMARY OF WORKSHOP 2

Lauren Hughes concluded the workshop by summarizing her takeaways from the presentations and discussions. She noted several speakers emphasized the importance of evidence-based community engagement at the individual, family, and community levels. She said community engagement should include co-creation, being inclusive, sharing governance, being culturally centered, and prioritizing building trust and trustworthiness.

Hughes said she learned from today's speakers that when performing data collection, researchers should consider the purpose of collecting the data, representativeness of the data collected, and whether that data matters to patients, clinicians, policy makers, and other stakeholders. She said speakers also highlighted the importance of developing a strategy to address incomplete data on race, ethnicity, and social risk factors. Speakers also suggested researchers should consider input from the end users of data regarding their data access and utilization needs. Speakers said partnerships and collaborations for data collection and use can play a major role in advancing PCOR. Speakers also suggested both building upon existing data infrastructure and building entirely new infrastructures to support new research methods, such as artificial intelligence.

Hughes noted that the discussion raised the importance of recruiting and developing an equity-minded research workforce. Speakers suggested research funders should consider requiring equity impact measurement in comparative effectiveness research. Speakers also said the extended time it currently takes to translate research findings into practice and to impact policy suggests a need to make translation and uptake an active and faster process rather than a passive one. Speakers also emphasized that the representativeness of the research sample used to develop an underlying body of evidence should be considered when disseminating and implementing new interventions and programs.

9

Workshop 3, Session 1: Measuring the Impact of Dissemination Projects

> **Key Messages Presented by Individual Speakers**
> - Researchers can gain useful insight by examining patient behaviors and health outcomes after the end of an implementation project. (Glanz)
> - Dissemination and implementation projects would benefit from creating more inclusive environments that engage faith-based and community-based organizations. The leaders of these organizations are embedded in underserved communities and are known and trusted by community members. (Buchanan)
> - Co-create community messaging materials and implementation strategies with community members. (Kwan)

WORKSHOP INTRODUCTION

Lauren Hughes, associate professor of family medicine and state policy director of the Farley Health Policy Center at the University of Colorado, offered brief introductory remarks. She explained that this workshop would focus on measuring the impact of dissemination and implementation projects. Karin Rhodes, the Agency for Healthcare Research and Quality (AHRQ) chief implementation officer, reviewed AHRQ's role related to the Patient-Centered

Outcomes Research Trust Fund (PCORTF) as well as their recent work related to developing and obtaining feedback about their strategic framework for priorities to guide their work. She then explained that AHRQ interpreted dissemination to include evidence generating, synthesis, translation, communication, assisting with implementing the evidence into clinical practice, and training. The presentations for this workshop were divided into two sessions with a speaker discussion held at the end of each discussion.

EVALUATING DISSEMINATION AND IMPLEMENTATION PROJECTS

Karen Glanz is the George A. Weiss University professor and professor in the Perelman School of Medicine and School of Nursing, associate director for community-engaged research, and program coleader for the cancer control program at the University of Pennsylvania Abramson Center. She discussed the many ways to measure the effectiveness of dissemination and implementation projects and determine which outcomes are most pertinent to stakeholders. Glanz began by discussing the Reach, Effectiveness, Adoption, Implementation, and Maintenance (RE-AIM) framework. The RE-AIM framework is an overarching structure for framing and evaluating the different dimensions or elements of implementation and dissemination research projects that investigators have used extensively for the past 20 years (Gaglio et al., 2013; Glasgow et al., 2019).

Glanz explained that a project she and her colleagues have been conducting for 24 years, called Pool Cool Field Research and Implementation, has generated practice-based evidence about implementation, maintenance, and sustainability. The project, aimed at skin cancer prevention, uses educational and environmental components, including signage, sunscreen, shade structures, and guidance for implementing sun-safe policies. After promising findings from a pilot program and subsequent clinical trial were published, the Centers for Disease Control and Prevention (CDC) encouraged Glanz and her collaborators to disseminate the program beyond the initial research sites. Between 2000 and 2002, her team conducted a pilot dissemination trial involving over 280 pools across the United States (Glanz et al., 2009). This was followed by a hybrid implementation and effectiveness trial at over 400 pools nationwide that ran from 2003 to 2008. As part of that trial, her team conducted a supplemental evaluation of the process used, as well as validation testing of the measures used (Glanz et al., 2010, 2015). This generated approximately 70,000 survey results (Escoffery et al., 2008; Hall et al., 2009).

Glanz continued to operate the Pool Cool website after the end of the study so any pool could reproduce and use the dissemination materials.[1]

---

[1] https://www.med.upenn.edu/poolcool (accessed September 14, 2022).

Glanz highlighted several lessons learned from that project that were applicable to community health programs, programs in health care settings, and others:

- Use all available types of measures.
- Be creative.
- Conduct more labor-intensive measures on a subsample of participants and sites.
- Long-term sustainability can be observed after the formal project has concluded and can serve as practice-based evidence.

Glanz said it is important for research to continue to observe patient behaviors and health outcomes after the implementation ends. This helps researchers identify and measure the outcomes most meaningful to stakeholders. She offered an example of a hypothetical study to evaluate outcomes of an implementation program related to primary care physicians and oncologists referring patients to evidence-based, effective treatment programs for tobacco dependence. She listed three possible outcomes that could be measured to evaluate implementation effectiveness: the number of patients given referrals, how many patients engage with the program immediately following the referral, and what level of cessation of tobacco use the patient ultimately achieves. The third outcome can only be measured if researchers continue observation after the end date of the implementation project.

USING DIGITAL TOOLS FOR DISSEMINATION AND IMPLELENTATION IN THE COMMUNITY

Silas Buchanan, founder and chief executive officer of the Institute for eHealth Equity, explained that his organization is a social impact consulting firm that works with people from underserved communities and communities of color to improve their digital literacy and to educate them about benefits of adopting and using technology to improve health outcomes. The organization also works with innovators in health technology to ensure that the solutions they develop are culturally responsive.

Buchanan said his organization crafts geographically expandable, web-based technology solutions that connect leaders of faith-based and community-based organizations to the people they serve. These leaders and their organizations are usually embedded in historically underserved communities. They are also known and trusted by members of those communities. Buchanan's organization seeks to create a more inclusive environment that engages faith-based and community-based organizations beyond those that are most visible or those that researchers engage with regularly to connect them with the patients, consumers, and congregants they serve as well as with health care providers, payers, policy makers, and academic stakeholders.

This work began with a 6-month pilot project called Text4Wellness, a healthy eating and active living campaign driven by text messages. This educational program used two-way, real-time text messaging to leverage relationships with faith- and community-based organizations. The project's goal was to demonstrate the potential of mobile health technology to reduce health disparities by consistently reaching and engaging people from underserved communities with critical health information.

The project also sought to develop an evidence base on the efficacy of mobile health interventions with targeted populations. That evidence base could serve as a catalyst for the development of new models for public–private partnerships for leveraging mobile health to reach and engage targeted populations. These goals aligned with the U.S. Department of Health and Human Services (DHHS) National Prevention Strategy recommendations to focus on people living in communities that have been made vulnerable, provide community members with the tools and information they need to make healthy choices, and promote positive social actions that support healthy decision making. Buchanan explained that a critical component of that project was developing relationships with community leaders that community members knew and trusted. He emphasized the importance of trust to the success of projects that seek to improve community health outcomes. His organization collected data related to engagement throughout the 6-month pilot program. The 6-month pilot program had 2,500 participants who received over 25,000 text messages and over 500 shared links to various resources. All of those participants completed the program and had a 43 percent response rate to the texted questions.

This project led to a partnership with Morehouse School of Medicine to create other web-based ecosystems to connect leaders of faith-based organizations and support their health ministries. Based on the success of this program, among others, that the Institute for eHealth Equity has piloted, Buchanan's team is preparing to launch ourhealthycommunity.com, designed to engage with community-based organizations and create connections with stakeholders from health care and health care research.

COMMUNITY ENGAGEMENT IN EVALUATING THE EFFECTIVENESS OF DISSEMINATION AND IMPLEMENTATION PROJECTS

Bethany Kwan is an associate professor and associate vice chair for research for the University of Colorado (CU) School of Medicine's Department of Emergency Medicine and the director of dissemination and implementation research at the Colorado Clinical and Translational Sciences Institute. She discussed the mAb Colorado project,[2] an implementation and real-world effectiveness study of monoclonal antibodies (mAbs) for high-risk outpatients with COVID-19. The three goals of this hybrid implementation and effectiveness study are to assess barriers and facilitators to using mAb infusion treatments statewide based on diffusion of innovations theory; develop, implement, and evaluate innovative strategies statewide to optimize equitable mAb access; and determine the real-world effectiveness and safety of mAb treatment in high-risk COVID-19 outpatients as new virus variants arise (Kwan et al., 2022b).

Kwan and her collaborators established a stakeholder advisory panel to develop a dissemination strategy for their study. They also held community engagement studios to codesign messages and materials for multiple audiences, including those for community-level messaging. The stakeholder panel, which included public health officials and representatives from different faith-based and community-based organizations, met twice a month for a year to ensure that all of the project's dissemination and implementation activities were designed to meet the needs of the community. Kwan's team also designed an implementation blueprint to provide a referral checklist for clinician-level effect.[3]

Kwan's team, when first engaging with the advisory panel, asked the panel members to identify their goals for the project. The most frequently cited goal was to achieve equitable access to care. The panel expressed concern about reaching people in Colorado's more rural areas, particularly given the distance rural residents would have to drive to reach an mAb infusion site. The panel believed this would reduce those patients' interest in receiving mAb therapy. The panel was also concerned about equitable access for people who are uninsured, underinsured, undocumented, or experiencing homelessness, as well as for people from minoritized racial and ethnic groups. Approximately one-quarter of Coloradans identify as Hispanic or Latino, said Kwan, and many only speak Spanish. There are also many people from Native American communities that live in Colorado. The project collaborated with people from those communities to develop culturally responsive materials specifically for those communities. The Colorado Health Institute, an informatics and data-based organization, created maps that Kwan's team used to assess effects at multiple levels over time throughout the project (Figure 9-1).

---

[2] Additional information is available at https://medschool.cuanschutz.edu/mab-colorado (accessed September 14, 2022).
[3] Available at https://medschool.cuanschutz.edu/docs/librariesprovider320/provider-page-library/mab-implementation-blueprint.pdf?sfvrsn=9080bcba_2 (accessed September 14, 2022).

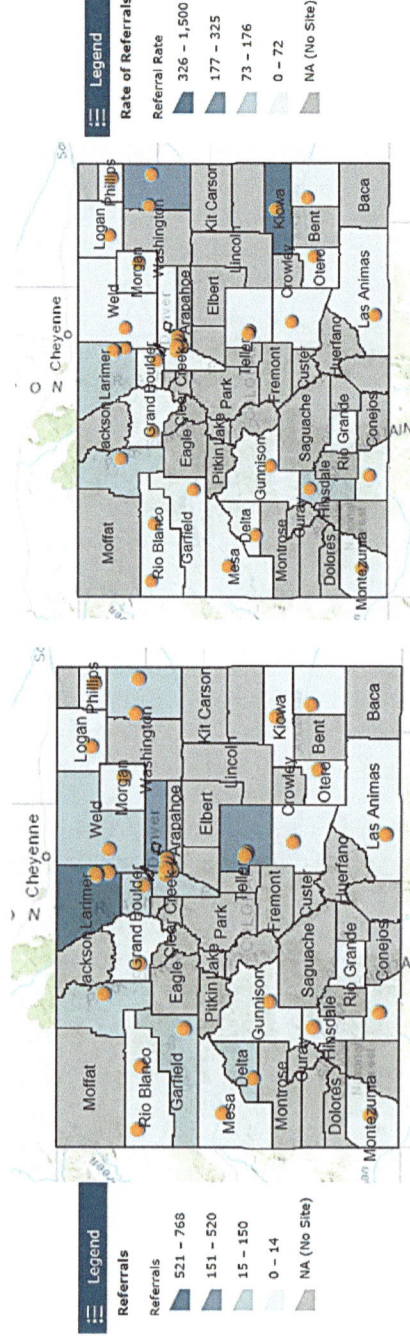

FIGURE 9-1 Total referrals (left) and referrals per 1,000 cases (right) for use of mAbs in Colorado as of July 31, 2021
NOTE: The orange dots indicate the location of infusion sites.
SOURCE: Adapted from the CU Monoclonal Antibody Referral Locations Web App (https://medschool.cuanschutz.edu/mab-colorado/research/mab-data-map). This work was supported by grant NIH/NCATS Colorado CTSA Grant Number UL1-TR002535-03 and 3UL1TR002535-03S3. Its contents are the authors' sole responsibility and do not necessarily represent official NIH views. Presented by Bethany Kwan on July 2, 2022, at Accelerating the Use of Findings from Patient-Centered Outcomes Research in Clinical Practice to Improve Health and Health Care: A Workshop Series.

DISCUSSION

Considerations for Community Engagement

Lauren Hughes's first question to the panelists asked them to identify key study infrastructure elements for engaging the community in evaluating the effectiveness of dissemination and implementation projects. Buchanan replied that bidirectional communication is critically important for ensuring that leaders of faith- and community-based organizations are effectively and authentically engaged. He noted that too frequently, researchers will begin outreach efforts to engage with a community after the project structure and budget have been created. As a result, community members do not have an opportunity to have input into a project that is about them. He added that it would be beneficial for researchers to share their results with the community in a format that the embedded faith- and community-based organizations can use to apply for their own grant funding. Those organizations may have been involved in providing or acquiring data for researchers funded by large grants. However, because those same organizations do not have quantitative or qualitative data for their community, their own grant applications are not as strong and they receive less funding. He also reiterated the important role that trust plays in encouraging leaders of faith- and community-based organizations to become involved in a project.

Glanz emphatically agreed with Buchanan's comment that having stakeholders involved from the start of a project is extremely important. She explained that an effective approach that her team uses at the initiation of a dissemination project is to seek opportunities for participants from community organizations to develop a sense of ownership for the project. As an example, she has found creating staff development opportunities for community organization staff, such as the lifeguards that participated in her project, was an effective strategy for developing a sense of ownership among members of the community. Her team also found community engagement studios to be valuable for developing a sense of community ownership of a project. She noted that this strategy has remained effective in a virtual format during the COVID-19 pandemic.

Kwan commented that the regional health connectors and practice-based research networks (PBRNs) serve as critical distribution channels into the community because of the strong relationships they have with their communities. She noted that developing productive relationships with these groups takes time, and one reason the mAb Colorado project was able to move so quickly was because she had long-term, well-established relationships with these organizations. Kwan also reiterated Buchanan's point that researchers should return data to the community in a form it can use for its own purposes.

Kwan, in responding to an audience request to discuss resources that describe how to establish and moderate community engagement studios, replied that the website dicemethods.org, run by the University of Colorado School of Medicine, has a list of community engagement methods. The list includes fact sheets and strategy guides for implementation of community engagement studios[4] and other engagement activities, both in person and virtually. She added that usually community engagement studios consist of two 90- to 120-minute sessions, held either in person or virtually. A community navigator and academic expert serve as moderators. The studio begins with a brief expert presentation describing the evidence that the project team will disseminate and the issues researchers are seeking to understand. That is followed by a discussion based on a series of two to three key codesign questions that will inform that development process.

Hughes asked Glanz to discuss possible approaches for engaging organizations in an accessible and sustainable manner to help them move toward evidence-based practice. Glanz replied that involving organizations that participate in the research phase of a project in the dissemination and implementation process is one approach that she has found effective. She added that a member of the community that embraces the process and acts as a local champion is also helpful. Glanz echoed Buchanan's comments, noting that building strong, trusting relationships is also necessary for developing a program that meets the community's needs and expectations. She added that this will also increase the likelihood that the organization will implement evidence-based practices that in turn will generate practice-based evidence.

Considerations for Research Funders

An audience member asked the panelists to comment on what role they see funders such as AHRQ playing in ensuring that the evaluation of dissemination and implementation projects involves community and patient stakeholders. Glanz replied that when her team was writing the proposal for a Patient-Centered Outcomes Research Institute (PCORI) Engagement Award, the application included rules that defined the amount of money that was required to be allocated to the community. She said that this may not be the most effective approach because it may limit the resources that the project can provide. She added that it is also important to consider fairness in the way a project team allocates resources among community partners and to avoid assuming that every community or organization has the same resource needs.

---

[4] Additional information is available at https://dicemethods.org/CENR (accessed September 14, 2022).

Kwan suggested that research funding agencies allow projects to use grant funds to purchase food for participants during community engagement activities. Some agencies have specific language in grant contracts barring the use of funds to purchase food for participants. She explained that while this seems like a minor consideration, it could improve the participant experience. She also suggested that applications should require inclusion of specific plans for active dissemination of research products back to the participants and the broader community in a form they can understand and use. Buchanan noted that monetary compensation is important. He suggested that a person that shares their time and data with a research project should receive more than food as reimbursement. He added that it is important to listen to community members in a manner that conveys that the project team values their contributions to the project and prioritizes making that data useful for the community. Kwan agreed that paying those who engage in planning and conducting research is critically important.

10

Workshop 3, Session 2: Measuring the Impact of Dissemination Projects Part 2

> **Key Messages Presented by Individual Speakers**
> - Enrolling non-representative trial sample groups that do not represent the full range of individuals in the target population can diminish external validity. This can lead to overestimating or underestimating what the effects of the dissemination and implementation project will be in the target population. (Stephens-Shields)
> - The Capability, Opportunity, and Motivation Model of Behavior (COM-B model) and the Normalization Process Theory model can serve as frameworks for developing effective dissemination and implementation programs for digital tools. (Politi)
> - Developing effective digital tools for health care is an iterative process, which may need greater consideration when designing funding for such projects. (Chaiyachati)

GENERALIZABILITY AND TEMPORALITY IN ASSESSING EFFECT

Alisa Stephens-Shields, associate professor of biostatistics at the University of Pennsylvania Perelman School of Medicine, discussed generalizability and temporality in assessing the effect of dissemination and implementation projects. Generalizability reflects the extent to which study findings apply to target populations. This requires minimizing discrepancies between study samples and target populations. Enrolling non-representative trial sample populations that do not represent the full range of individuals in the target population can diminish external validity. This can lead to overestimating or underestimating what the effects of the dissemination and implementation project will be in the target population.

She then discussed the Randomized Evaluation of Trial Acceptance by Incentive (RETAIN) trial that she conducted with colleagues at the University of Pennsylvania. This trial, explained Stephens-Shields, evaluated financial incentives as a means of recruiting sufficient participants to increase representativeness and generate generalizable trial results. It also explored the ethics of using incentives to increase enrollment. The study investigated whether financial incentives lead to "undue inducement" that disproportionately increased enrollment among people from systematically divested communities. She added that undue inducement is an incentive that blunts the perceived risk of participating in the trial or an incentive that is unjust.

Graphic representation of data indicating undue inducement is characterized by a difference in the slope of the relationship of perceived riskiness and the probability of enrollment according to the size of the incentive (Figure 10-1). She explained that when there is no incentive, people will be less likely to enroll in a trial if they believe it is risky. However, if paying the participants increases the probability of enrollment for the same amount of perceived risk, this reflects undue inducement. Similarly, a large difference in the slope of enrollment versus incentive size according to economic status is reflective of unjust inducement (Figure 10-2).

Stephens-Shields then discussed the Behavioral Economics to Transform Trial Enrollment Representativeness (BETTER) project, an initiative funded by the American Heart Association to test behavioral economics interventions. The study seeks to determine whether behavioral economics interventions are an effective mechanism to surmount the barriers to randomized controlled trial participation faced by people from disenfranchised racial and ethnic groups, women, people with low incomes, or people with a medical risk of cardiovascular disease. A key target outcome for BETTER is achieving an increase in the enrollment fraction. This represents the number of individuals enrolled out of the number of individuals from different subgroups who are contacted to participate in a trial. The primary outcome for BETTER's second component will be the enrollment fraction of Black and Latino participants. She noted that the study has identified them as important subgroups that are disproportionately affected by adverse cardiovascular health outcomes but are less likely to enroll in cardiovascular health clinical trials. A secondary out-

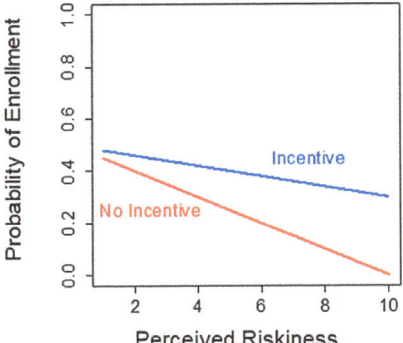

FIGURE 10-1 A large difference in the slope of the enrollment versus risk relationship indicates that the incentive results in undue inducement (graph is for illustrative purposes and does not represent data from an actual study)
SOURCE: Presented by Alisa Stephens-Shields on July 1, 2022, at Accelerating the Use of Findings from Patient-Centered Outcomes Research in Clinical Practice to Improve Health and Health Care: A Workshop Series.

come will examine the enrollment fraction overall stratified by socioeconomic status. The project will also measure the population to prevalence ratio—the enrollment fraction of specific subgroups divided by the overall enrollment fraction—to determine whether the intervention produces more representative samples. This measure will also enable researchers to determine the true

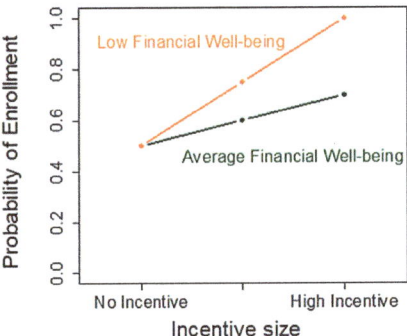

FIGURE 10-2 A large difference in the slope of the enrollment versus incentive size according to economic status indicates that the incentive results in unjust inducement (graph is for illustrative purposes and does not represent data from an actual study)
SOURCE: Presented by Alisa Stephens-Shields on July 1, 2022, at Accelerating the Use of Findings from Patient-Centered Outcomes Research in Clinical Practice to Improve Health and Health Care: A Workshop Series.

population effect in the target populations and examine heterogeneity among different socioeconomic and racial groups.

Stephens-Shields and her collaborators are assessing the sequential effect of an intervention using the mediation framework to examine temporality (Baron and Kenny, 1986). This framework involves measuring the direct effect of an intervention on an outcome versus the outcome when the intervention goes through a mediator. The mediation framework proved important for determining why an intervention did not work in a trial that aimed to increase condom use by African American men who had sex with men (Jemmott et al., 2015). That study found two theoretical constructs that were strongly associated with condom usage that the intervention did not affect: a negotiation skill and peer descriptive norms. As a result, the study investigators designed future interventions to target those two constructs.

In closing, Stephens-Shields provided some questions that these studies highlight related to assessing effect. Those include the following:

- How well do the data used to evaluate the effect reflect the population in which we want to apply conclusions, and how can we minimize relevant gaps?
- Are thresholds and benchmarks used in evaluating the effect meaningful?
- Have we generated sufficient longitudinal data to assess sequences of effect and provide insight into the mechanism of effect or lack thereof?

CLINICIAN ENGAGEMENT WITH A BREAST RECONSTRUCTION DECISION SUPPORT TOOL

Mary Politi, professor of surgery at Washington University in St. Louis School of Medicine, discussed clinician engagement with decision support tools using a breast reconstruction digital support tool project she collaborated on as an example. The project involved a diverse group of stakeholders and researchers from Washington University in St. Louis and the Ohio State University. These included decision scientists; plastic and reconstructive surgeons; an infectious disease expert who studied complications from breast reconstruction; and individuals with expertise in clinical informatics, data analysis, data management, and research administration. The project's stakeholder advisory group included patient partners from varying regions of the country; surgeons from varying regions of the country; and informatics specialists who helped with the logistics of incorporating the tool into the electronic health record (EHR). Both groups worked to guide the tool development and implementation process.

Politi and her colleagues piloted the first version of a breast reconstruction decision support tool in an earlier randomized trial. They compared the decision tool to enhanced usual care and found that patients in the intervention group were more knowledgeable about the risks and benefits of the different options related to breast reconstruction (Politi et al., 2020). They also found that patients also had a slightly higher, though not statistically significant, decision process quality; patients reported increased certainty about their choice; and patients were more actively engaged in their care. An important finding from this study was that the intervention (the decision support tool) had no effect on consultation length. That indicated that the decision support tool did not affect clinical workflows, an important factor to the participating clinicians. However, after the study, clinicians reported that at times they were unsure whether a patient had used the tool, which affected their engagement with the patient. Politi explained that the clinicians wanted to use the tool to engage in shared decision making, which became the goal of a subsequent implementation project.

Politi and her collaborators relied on the Capability, Opportunity, and Motivation Model of Behavior (COM-B model) as a framework for understanding behavior change as they began considering their approach to facilitating clinician engagement with the decision support tool. They identified four required elements for clinicians to change their behavior (engage with the tool):

1. the capability to use the tool, which requires skills and training;
2. motivation to use the tool, which requires believing it will help the clinical encounter and may also involve incentivizing use;
3. opportunities to use the tool, which requires resources and possibly integrating the tool into the EHR; and
4. social norms, such as the perception that their peers are using the tool and finding it beneficial.

Politi also described another implementation framework that she has found to be effective: Normalization Process Theory (Hooker et al., 2015; Hooker and Taft, 2016; Toye, 2016). This process identifies four important components of implementation:

1. coherence, or defining the work, its benefits, and how it will affect the clinician's practice;
2. cognitive participation, or who does the work and what are the teams involved in implementation;
3. collective action, or how the work gets done and what is needed for the intervention to become part of routine care; and
4. reflexive monitoring, or how the clinician understands the work and what the effect will be in terms of measured outcomes.

Politi then described the BREASTChoice breast reconstruction decision support tool and the process of developing it through the lens of those models. She began with their approach to addressing coherence. Patients initially receive access to the web-based breast reconstruction decision tool, which describes the different options for breast reconstruction, via the patient portal for their physician's EHR or email. The tool includes educational modules that address whether to have breast reconstruction; types of reconstruction procedures; timing and risk for each type of procedure; and reconstruction outcome photos.

Politi explained that in terms of coherence and cognitive participation, there was minimal work required on the part of clinicians to use the tool at her institution. Politi noted that all of the pertinent clinicians at both institutions completed the training and were supportive of the tool. The decision support tool was integrated into their EHR. Clinicians could access the tool's summary by clicking an icon below a patient's name. At Ohio State the process was less streamlined. Clinicians were required to first click a button in the EHR to agree to add the tool and summary, followed by clicking another to allow the data to be imported into the patient chart in the EHR.

Next, Politi addressed the cognitive participation and collective action component. The researchers were required to send the enrollment link for the decision support tool to patients who consented via the MyChart patient portal or email. Schedulers from the clinician's office could also send flyers to eligible patients that explained they would be contacted by a member of the clinical team prior to using the tool. Surgical oncologists received flyers that they could provide to their patients prior to a referral to a plastic and reconstructive surgeon.

Politi next elaborated on their application of the COM-B model. The clinicians were provided training to develop skills for using the decision support tool. The research team found that some clinicians lacked motivation to use the tool. However, the tool was automated, so clinicians were required to do little work to use it. She noted that the COVID-19 pandemic prevented the research staff from being in the clinic to observe workflow during usability testing. One surprising finding was that many clinicians were comfortable with the paper printout, which the research team did not expect given that it was a digital tool.

Politi described some of the challenges the researchers encountered related to physician engagement with the decision-making tool. While many clinicians were accustomed to viewing information in the EHR, they were less acclimated to doing so in the context of shared decision making with a patient. Some clinicians were comfortable sending information to patients for them to review. However, the researchers had to put forth substantial effort to move the clinicians to use that information to support collaborative decision making with the patient. Another challenge to clinician engagement was finding solutions to address EHR alert fatigue. Politi noted that further research is needed to ascertain optimal design for the tool, including how best to provide alerts. Other subjects for future research include determining how to integrate clinician components into patient-facing tools; investigating the role of EHR restrictions, institution policies, and culture in the effectiveness of the decision support tool; how to build on existing workflows and engage clinical champions; and investigating whether integrating engagement with decision support tools into resident training would increase clinician engagement.

INCORPORATING PCOR INTO CLINICAL PRACTICE: A DIGITAL TECHNOLOGY CASE STUDY

Krisda Chaiyachati, physician lead for value-based care and innovation at Verily Health Platforms and adjunct senior fellow at the University of Pennsylvania's Leonard Davis Institute of Health Economics, began by remarking that he is pleased to observe the growing emphasis on accelerating how social science, behavioral science, and health services research are making it into clinical practice and touching patients' lives. He also acknowledged that this will be a challenging process. Chaiyachati said that there are innumerable ways in which digital technology interacts with the health care system (Figure 10-3), illustrated by the many digital tools already in use or in development (Abernethy et al., 2022). This has resulted in a large variety of stakeholders in the digital transformation of health and health care that are affected by decisions related to dissemination and implementation. This includes small technology startups, large technology firms, academia, health care delivery organizations, regulators, patients, and communities. He echoed Buchanan, noting that the growth of digital technologies in health care has implications for equity and inclusivity.

Chaiyachati next recounted a story from his perspective about the beginning of the COVID-19 pandemic. In March 9, 2020, he and a colleague were in Philadelphia watching news coverage of COVID-19 as it began to spread globally. At the time, there were reports of alarming conditions in northern Italy, cruise ships carrying people that had been infected with COVID-19 were not allowed to dock, and intensive care units (ICUs) were beginning to overflow in Seattle and New York City. While hospitals in Philadelphia had not yet been overwhelmed by patients with COVID-19, staff had become concerned owing to the increasing number of scared people calling or coming to the Penn Health system's emergency departments. This prompted the formation of a large team at Penn Health to cultivate strategies to address the challenge of identifying people infected with SARS-CoV-2 and which patients required hospitalization.

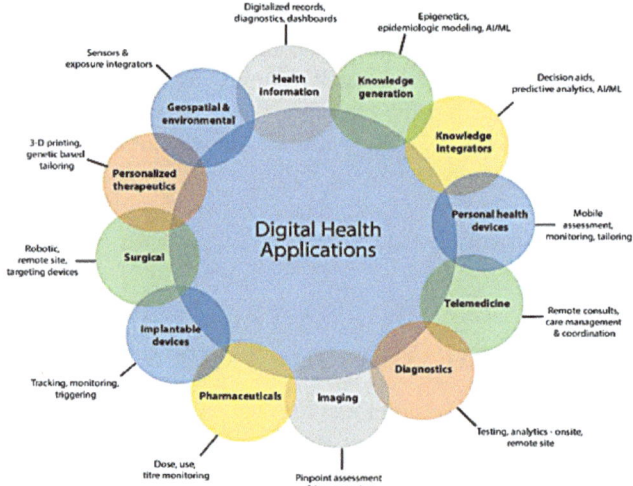

FIGURE 10-3 Evolving applications of digital technology in health and health care
NOTE: AI/ML = artificial intelligence and machine learning.
SOURCE: Reproduced from the National Academy of Medicine publication *The Promise of Digital Health: Then, Now, and the Future* (2022). Presented by Krisda Chaiyachati on July 2, 2022, at Accelerating the Use of Findings from Patient-Centered Outcomes Research in Clinical Practice to Improve Health and Health Care: A Workshop Series (Abernathy et al., 2022).

The team at Penn was seeking to decrease the likelihood of their emergency departments being overwhelmed by developing a mechanism to ensure patients with serious illness were brought to the emergency department and those that did not require that level of care did not present to the emergency department. Chaiyachati explained that was the first design consideration for developing a useful digital tool. The second consideration was that COVID-19 was presenting with a variety of symptoms, but the associated respiratory failure and COVID pneumonia appeared to be resulting in fatalities. Chaiyachati and his colleagues designed a digital tool that could identify patients who were developing shortness of breath because that had been identified as a symptom associated with poor disease outcome. The result was a text message–based program called COVID Watch (Morgan et al., 2020). COVID Watch sent text message check-ins twice daily, in either English or Spanish, that asked individuals about their shortness of breath and if they found breathing more difficult than usual. The system would automatically connect the individual, depending on their responses, to a team of telemedicine providers who were available 24 hours a day.

Chaiyachati noted that the team engaged in substantial observation and experimentation that occurred prior to determining the final design of the program (Morgan et al., 2020). Chaiyachati ran a randomized controlled trial testing whether supplementing patient responses with objective pulse oximetry improved outcomes. However, he found that this approach did not affect outcomes (Lee et al., 2022). The design team also interviewed patients regarding their experience using the program. The team continued to modify COVID Watch as they received feedback. Chaiyachati noted an informal study conducted a comparison of COVID Watch with a similar program at Northwestern University. The Northwestern University program relied on manual enrollment and was staffed by registered nurses between 8 a.m. and 8 p.m. The study found that COVID Watch saved Penn Medicine about $2.3 million every 100 days. That benefit accrued because COVID Watch was automated and thus only required 64 staff hours per day compared with 500 hours required for the Northwestern program. Patient satisfaction for COVID Watch had a 90 net promotor score, which Chaiyachati said is comparable to the score that Apple products receive. The program also achieved a relative reduction of mortality of 64 percent (Delgado et al., 2021). In addition, COVID Watch was able to manage patient volumes efficiently, differentiate patients who required evaluation in the emergency department, and effectively monitor those individuals that did not require evaluation in the emergency department.

Chaiyachati noted that more than 30 individuals were involved in creating COVID Watch. This highlighted the complexity of designing a robust program that integrates with existing technology, engages the clinical team, and enables the research evaluation needed to generate supporting evidence. He explained that there is a need to find balance between the quality and the rigor needed to generate evidence and the ability to scale and spread innovations such as this or create parallel models in other disease conditions. Chaiyachati said that in the future, digital health tools should be designed with the capability to account for a patient's entire life span, the variety of physical and emotional conditions that can affect them, and the effect of social determinants of health. He closed by summarizing insights he gained during the process of developing COVID Watch. He discussed lessons the team learned during the COVID Watch project. He said that digital health tools can enhance human-powered care. The efficiency of care provided with the support of digital health tools affects the degree to which patients and providers are receptive to using the tool. It is important to ensure equity and define the measures of equity early in the intervention design process. He encouraged funders to support the design stage and not focus solely on outcomes because the design of digital health interventions is critical for successful implementation and uptake.

DISCUSSION

Behavioral Economics

Session moderator Sarah Scholle, vice president for research and analysis at the National Committee for Quality Assurance (NCQA), posed an audience question to Stephens-Shields that asked her to discuss how the principles of behavioral economics can help improve implementation, dissemination, and sustained use of evidence-based interventions. Stephens-Shields explained that behavioral economics is an important component of effective dissemination and implementation because frequently evidence of effectiveness is not an adequate stimulus for people to change or adopt a new behavior. Behavioral economics provides a useful tool to inform and adjust implementation and dissemination efforts to frame outcomes as rewards versus relying on loss aversion as a source of motivation. She noted that she is just starting a new program that will use nudging techniques, a standard approach in behavioral economics, in a telemedicine setting to encourage patients to follow up on care, such as completing recommended screening tests following identification of an irregularity during a clinical marker.

Chaiyachati agreed that behavioral economics can offer critical insights into how to use people's innate, often irrational behaviors to move them toward their desired health goals. He suggested that there are opportunities to blend behavioral health economics with social science, implementation science, statistics, and other fields to accelerate the process of translating research discoveries into clinical practices. Behavioral economics principles can be tested with small changes during the preparation phase; such tests can be done quickly in a small trial, which can reduce delays during the later stages of determining a final design. Chaiyachati said that it would be economically advantageous to fund this newer approach of rapid testing and iteration and integrate it into randomized controlled trials. He suggested that this approach could support innovation by allowing academic researchers to feel less constrained when designing a new tool. He added that industry already uses this approach in its implementation and dissemination research. Stephens-Shields commented that being adaptive during the research process implies changing as more information accrues while still following established principles.

When asked how this approach would allow interventions to address the needs of different patients and populations, Stephens-Shields said there are enrichment designs for clinical trials that allow some interim preliminary evaluation of whether an intervention is more promising in certain subgroups than others. This allows the trial to pivot enrollment strategies to target those promising groups. Chaiyachati added that different communities have different preferences for the manner in which they interact with the health care system and those preferences change over time. He noted that while research might examine individual behaviors and preferences among specific subgroups, it can create operational challenges if an iterative process results in creating multiple different profiles and multiple different operational programs for different types of people. He added that additional research is needed to determine how to do this effectively.

Considering Metrics

Scholle asked the panelists to discuss potential metrics that would provide Agency for Healthcare Research and Quality (AHRQ) insights into optimal strategies for engaging different populations in research as well as the scalability of various interventions. Stephens-Shields replied that some of the metrics her team is using in the BETTER project relate to the engagement of different demographic groups in research. These include enrollment fraction and population prevalence ratios that allow for gauging the representativeness of a sample. She added that universal application of these types of metrics would be useful for gaining an understanding of the research landscape versus the landscape for a specific project.

Chaiyachati said metrics that are applied across patient populations and across delivery organizations would provide information about equity and the inequities that might occur with an intervention. This is not something that AHRQ has explicitly asked research communities to consider when an intervention targets a population that has traditionally had challenges accessing care. He suggested that another type of metric for AHRQ to consider would examine the spread of an implemented intervention beyond the primary institution or from clinic to clinic within the same health care system. This would assess the ability of an intervention to spread and scale to neighboring health care systems. This would be particularly germane given the challenges that arise from a lack of interoperable data systems, both within a health care system and between different health care systems.

Considering Stakeholders

Scholle asked the panelists to discuss their ideas for how AHRQ might consider the perspectives of different stakeholders and different resources, whether it is data or workflow, as a means of improving scalability and broader spread of interventions. Chaiyachati began by noting that the amount of data that could be used in health care is growing rapidly and substantially. He expressed concern that health system data infrastructure may not be able to process and manage all of that data. Additionally, some health care systems may not be able to bear the cost of processing and managing this large volume of data. He noted this could be particularly challenging for those practices or health care systems that are not part of large academic medical centers. He suggested that funders should consider whether they could support health care systems to address these challenges.

Scholle asked the group to discuss possible strategies to address alert fatigue that may interfere with the effectiveness of nudges or other tools designed to draw a clinician's attention. Stephens-Shields said researchers can build measures for responsiveness into an intervention trial to identify where and when diminishing returns occur related to frequency and extent of nudging. She added that researchers should be conscious of the potential for alert fatigue and incorporate constructs to evaluate and address it into intervention trials. Chaiyachati then suggested incorporating de-implementation science[1] to determine when it is appropriate to turn off certain alerts and which alerts are most critical to retain. He added this is particularly critical to the ICU setting. He then offered an example from his experience as a general internist. At times when he initially opens a patient chart in the EHR, he encounters 15–20 alerts or reminders for tasks to complete during that clinical encounter. He suggested further research into approaches to optimize context and timing for those alerts. He also suggested that an EHR alert for a clinician may not be the optimal solution. Another approach could be to develop a system that delivers this information to patients, encouraging them to take a more active role in their health care.

Resource Considerations

Stephens-Shields also responded to Scholle's question about generalizability and what would be necessary to implement an intervention in settings with different resources. Stephens-Shields highlighted the importance of inclusive research and recruitment strategies that include health care systems in different settings with different levels of infrastructure and other resources. This strategy will assist developers to gain an understanding of the limitations on potential effects in certain settings and identify additional supports certain systems might need to implement an intervention and achieve the desired outcomes. She also suggested that AHRQ should consider investing in the infrastructure that would allow health care systems to manage and process large volumes of data.

Chaiyachati added that artificial intelligence and machine learning (AI/

---

[1] De-implementation science identifies problem areas of low-value and wasteful practice, carries out rigorous scientific examination of the factors that initiate and maintain such behaviors, and then employs evidence-based interventions to cease these practices (Davidson et al., 2017).

ML) technology could support efforts to manage and analyze large amounts of data. He also emphasized the need to ensure that AI/ML do not perpetuate biases. Stephens-Shields echoed Chaiyachati regarding the need to address the issue of automated algorithms and equity.

Speakers' Closing Thoughts

To conclude the discussion, Scholle asked the panelists for any final thoughts regarding the most important things that would be beneficial for AHRQ to consider related to evaluating the effectiveness of its implementation and dissemination projects. Chaiyachati replied that from his perspective, there is a need to move beyond individual tests and the practice level and consider scalability and spread across multiple health systems. One approach would be to dedicate funding to specifically support scalability research and development of infrastructure that would better enable scalability and spread. Stephens-Shields said that while there are many different dimensions by which to measure and evaluate dissemination effects, inclusiveness is a key dimension. She also suggested evaluating implementation and dissemination projects across multiple stages.

CLOSING SUMMARY OF WORKSHOP 3

Lauren Hughes concluded the workshop by summarizing her takeaways from the presentations and discussions.

She described several suggestions made by speakers for incorporating community engagement into effective dissemination and implementation projects:[2]

- Engaging with a variety of community stakeholders to gain novel insight when conducting dissemination and implementation research.
- Involving community members early in the dissemination and implementation project planning process, and continuing engagement throughout the course of the project.
- Acknowledging the contributions of communities who have shared valuable data and perspectives by providing them with results in accessible forms so that they can use the findings to apply for funding themselves.

---

[2] These points were made by the individual workshop speakers/participants identified above. They are not intended to reflect a consensus among workshop participants.

Hughes also described speaker suggestions for developing effective dissemination and implementation projects. These included[3]

- Developing strategies to address the need for infrastructure that will enable researchers and clinicians to access to the rapidly growing amount of health care;
- Supporting dissemination of research results beyond presentations at academic conferences;
- Leveraging behavioral economic insights to support dissemination and implementation efforts;
- Considering the use of digital health tools and technologies to enhance health equity, personalize health care, and increase the efficiency of care;
- Examining how rigid structures and workflows may impede progress; and
- Learning from how other industries innovate.

---

[3] These points were made by the individual workshop speakers/participants identified above. They are not intended to reflect a consensus among workshop participants.

11

Workshop 4, Session 1: Effective Communication Tools

> **Key Messages Presented by Individual Speakers**
> - Effective communication of patient-centered outcomes must occur beyond research and academic communities. (Sharma)
> - It would be beneficial to integrate education about communicating longitudinally and outside of the formal success measure of journal publication in medical school and public policy graduate programs to improve translation of PCOR evidence to nonmedical audiences. (Sharma)
> - Some communities are in a constant state of crisis, which makes it challenging to communicate about health-related issues with them through the noise, unrest, and social inequities that are affecting those communities. (Ponder)
> - Information must be easily accessible for patients, providers, payers, and advocates to reduce barriers to being an informed consumer of health care. (Ponder)
> - Effective use of research findings to inform, persuade, and move people to action should include steps to engage people around issues that matter to them, understand their data needs and research priorities, and educate them about how a law or policy action may specifically affect them. (Hunter)
> - It is important to have a multifaceted legal and policy approach to advance health equity. (Hunter)

WORKSHOP INTRODUCTION

Lauren Hughes opened the final virtual workshop in the workshop series by noting that the day's presentations would focus on effective communication tools and informing evidence-based policy making. Karin Rhodes explained that historically, the Agency for Healthcare Research and Quality's (AHRQ's) role has been to disseminate evidence to health care stakeholders. It does this by synthesizing evidence from patient-centered outcomes research (PCOR) and across government agencies and then translating it and communicating it using various tools and decision support aids. AHRQ also helps practices implement evidence-based interventions into clinical practice and provides various training programs for clinicians. These activities are all consistent with AHRQ's congressional authorization to support the dissemination of evidence into practice and train the next generation of patient-centered outcomes researchers. Based on its first 10 years of work and current administration priorities, AHRQ has established a small set of priority areas on which it will focus its investments. Those areas are prevention and improved care of patients with chronic conditions; improving patient and family and provider experience of care to enhance trust in the health care system; promoting high-value, safe care that is aligned with national health priorities, which can change over time; and primary care transformation.

TRANSLATING POLICY AND PATIENT-CENTERED OUTCOMES OUTSIDE THE INSTITUTIONAL BUBBLE

Manisha Sharma, cofounder and chief strategy officer for CentiVox Media Group, began by explaining that one of the major barriers for communicating patient-centered outcomes effectively is that while the research and academic communities like to see practical uses of their research, those communities tend to limit communications regarding their research findings to the academic and research settings. This contributes to the current scenario of a large amount of data, science, and other information that is available but not always communicated effectively. Communities may be skeptical of the messengers who typically convey this information and who may not be the individuals that conducted the research. This skepticism creates opportunities for misinformation and disinformation to fill the resulting communication gaps and create confusion within the community. It also raises the critical question of how people perceive and receive communication.

Sharma explained that in 2020, during the height of the COVID-19 pandemic, Pew Research Center conducted a study to investigate which sources people were using to obtain news about the pandemic and the research being conducted to combat COVID-19 (Shearer and Mitchell, 2021; Shearer, 2021).

This study found that 86 percent of U.S. adults relied on digital sources, with Facebook serving as a regular source of that news for nearly one-third of U.S. adults. Sharma suggested that one barrier to progress is that the research community and the agencies that fund research frequently do not adequately engage with nonmedical and nonhealth audiences through the mediums they rely on for information. This is usually not within the confines of institutional walls or academic journals. Sharma, who is a board-certified family medicine physician, noted that frequently physician training conditions future physicians to place the responsibility of being well informed and health care literate on the consumer.

She explained that while there is a great deal of passion about conducting research that can advance health and health care within the research community, members of that community are unaware that the same passion exists among people outside of the traditional research community. Examples include community-based organizations, the patient advocacy space, and nongovernmental organizations. She noted that media platforms often rely on digital platforms and social media for information instead of journal publications or other sources typically used by researchers to communication findings. In addition, there is a generational change in how people perceive and receive news. While print media is still important for individuals aged 50 and older, digital media is increasing rapidly as an important source of information for younger U.S. adults (Shearer, 2021).

Sharma suggested additional efforts should be directed to train experts, starting in medical school and public policy graduate programs, in communicating longitudinally and outside of journal publications. She encouraged AHRQ to intentionally seek, prioritize, and fund researchers and research that are relatable, reliable, and effective. Her third suggestion was for AHRQ to build a diversity, equity, inclusion, and belonging workforce of people within the research community that includes people in leadership positions. She also suggested development of public relations strategies that include considering effective strategies for translating research by involving cross-sector collaborators who can help the communications department translate research findings into information that is meaningful to the target community or communities.

PERSPECTIVES IN HEALTH COMMUNICATION

Monica Ponder, assistant professor of health communication and culture in the Cathy Hughes School of Communications at Howard University, began by explaining that some communities are in a constant state of crisis, which makes it challenging to communicate about health-related issues with them through the noise, unrest, and social inequities that are affecting those communities (Ponder, 2022).

Health communication, explained Ponder, is the science and art of using communication to advance the health and well-being of people and populations. It is a multidisciplinary field of study that brings together evidence, strategy, theory, and creativity to promote behaviors, policies, and practices that advance the health and well-being of people and populations. Health communication, she noted, starts by focusing on the physician–patient relationship.

She explained that the public health pyramid (Figure 11-1) illustrates that achieving an increasing population effect requires several levels of interventions on which to focus (Frieden, 2010). For example, while counseling and education may work at the individual level, population change and population effects require environmental and structural approaches to public health. She added that health care is a continuum. Therefore, the goal of health communication should not be to reach people at the point of diagnosis, but at the point where promotion of health and prevention of disease is possible. This includes addressing policy and environmental levers and shifting collective behavior before people reach a state of distress. It is important that communications reflect an ecological approach that includes both individuals and

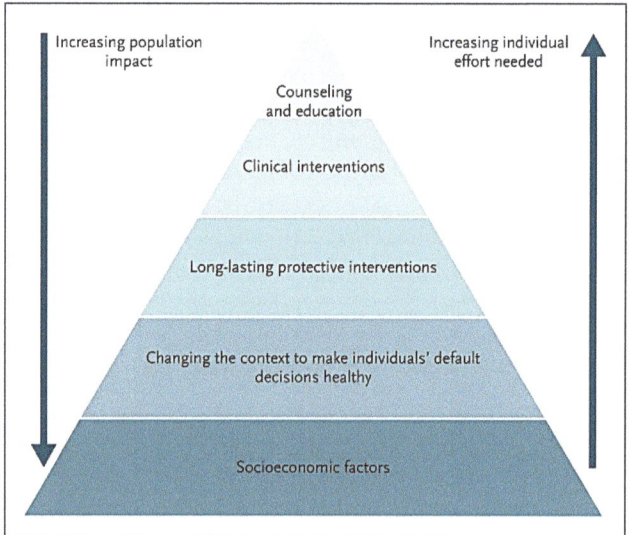

FIGURE 11-1 The public health impact pyramid
SOURCE: Adapted from Frieden, T. R. A framework for public health action: the health impact pyramid (2010), with permission from Sheridan. Presented by Monica Ponder on July 6, 2022, at Accelerating the Use of Findings from Patient-Centered Outcomes Research in Clinical Practice to Improve Health and Health Care: A Workshop Series.

health system partners. Communication efforts should also acknowledge that people are not only navigating multiple crises but are also receiving information from multiple sources that can intentionally or unintentionally counter the messages that health communication seeks to promote. Health literacy is an important tool to address these challenges because it gives people the capacity to obtain, process, and understand basic health information. Health literacy is important, she added, because low health literacy is linked to many adverse outcomes that burden both the individual and the health care system.

Ponder explained that communication can

- increase knowledge and awareness of a health issue, problem, or solution;
- influence perceptions, beliefs, and attitudes that may change social norms;
- advocate a position on a health issue or policy;
- increase demand or support for health services;
- refute myths and misconceptions; and
- strengthen organizational relationships.

There are structural issues, said Ponder, that communication cannot solve despite committed effort. This includes the ability to make sustained change or compensate for inadequate access to health care. Communications cannot produce sustained change in complex health behaviors without the support of a larger program for change, including components addressing health care services, technology, and changes in regulations and policy. She noted that communications may not be equally effective in addressing all issues or relaying all messages because of any of the following challenges: the topic or suggested behavior change may be complex, the intended audience may have preconceptions about the topic or messenger, or the topic may be controversial. She said the National Cancer Institute has produced a useful resource that explains what communication can and cannot do and provides examples of effective health communication approaches (National Cancer Institute, 2004).

Ponder said that when engaging in a communications project, it is important to center community voices in terms of their experiences and apply an ecological approach to understand social determinants and the structural elements that affect how people perceive and access information. It is also important for people to feel heard, that institutions are listening to them and that their input is valued. As an example, Ponder referred workshop attendees to visit the Project REFOCUS website.[1]

---

[1] Available at www.projectrefocus.com (accessed September 14, 2022).

HOW LAW AND POLICY CAN ADVANCE HEALTH EQUITY

Dawn Hunter, the Network for Public Health Law's southeastern region director, explained that her organization provides legal technical assistance, consulting, trainings, and resources to local, state, and national health agencies and organizations across the United States. Hunter and her colleagues work with public health leaders, policy makers, researchers, educators, advocates, and health care providers through no-cost legal technical assistance in the form of strategic consultation, knowledge building, research and analysis, and awareness building and connection.

Hunter's particular areas of specialization are the use of legal and policy strategies to promote health and racial equity, the structure and governance of public health agencies, and civic engagement as a health equity strategy. Hunter added that budgets are an important policy tool because a budget communicates values. Communication combined with law can play an important role in fomenting advocacy that engages communities and builds political will. However, she added, the legal community would benefit from improving efforts around communicating about the role of law and policy in shaping health outcomes.

Hunter said that there are many ways to use research, data, and storytelling to inform, persuade, and move people to action. The first part of this process requires engaging people around issues that reflect their priorities, understand their data needs and research priorities, and educate them about how a law or policy action could specifically affect them. The next step is the process of equipping people with the tools to engage with policy makers. That includes providing people with information and training them on how to use it effectively to mobilize around the community's priorities and take action. Examples of key mobilization actions, Hunter said, include contacting legislators, writing opinion pieces, working with a newspaper or news outlet on a story about a health issue in the community, or going to city council meetings. Then the effect of this work should be evaluated and the lessons learned applied to future efforts.

Hunter explained that there are other approaches to affect state-level policy through the legislative process. The process of drafting legislation is influenced by available research and data. This data is usually delivered by businesses, lobbyists, executive agencies, community advocates, and researchers, all of whom are communicating about something that is a priority to them. Her organization's recent survey of legislative trends over the last two legislative cycles found that almost every state has introduced a bill that affects health or racial equity. Trends that proposed legislation encompass include continuing efforts to address racism as a public health crisis or emergency, addressing educational inequities, prohibiting teaching of divisive concepts in schools, improving racial equity in state agency employments, data collection and use, and provider education and training. Other legislative trends were providing the infrastructure and funding to conduct health and racial equity work; addressing equity in birth outcomes, maternal, and child health broadly; and using racial equity or health impact statements in policy making. This last trend, said Hunter, is informed by the evidence on the need for conducting those types of assessments and in using evidence to conduct the assessment itself.

Hunter described examples of how the Five Essential Public Health Law Services framework connects with the AHRQ strategic framework to guide PCOR investments (Figure 11-2). Access to evidence and expertise informs needed policy changes, while expertise in designing and selecting legal and policy solutions enables disseminating evidence to health care decision makers. Implementing, enforcing, and defending local and national policy solutions will accelerate the uptake of evidence into practice and policy surveillance, Hunter said, and evaluation will tie into building data measurement and analytic capability. Hunter concluded by emphasizing the following: there are many ways to affect law and many types of law to affect, it is important to develop a multifaceted legal and policy approach to advance health equity, and strategic advocacy and communication are useful means of changing law and policy.

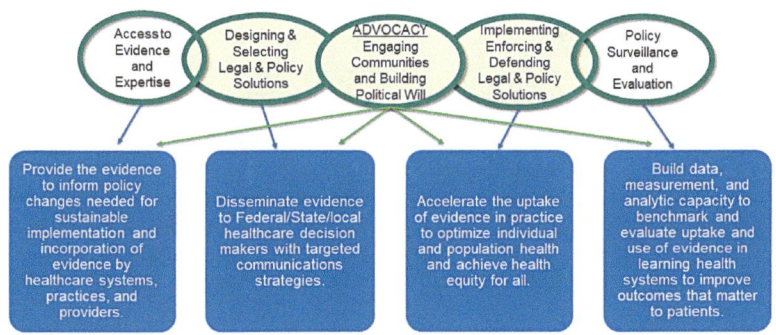

FIGURE 11-2 The role of law in advancing AHRQ's crosscutting strategies
SOURCE: Adapted from the 5 Essential Public Health Law Services model of the Network for Public Health Law (networkforphl.org). Presented by Dawn Hunter on July 6, 2022, at Accelerating the Use of Findings from Patient-Centered Outcomes Research in Clinical Practice to Improve Health and Health Care: A Workshop Series.

DISCUSSION

Tailoring Communication for the Audience

Session moderator Cara Nikolajski posed a question from audience member Grace Scharf, New York City Health and Hospitals, that asked the panelists for suggestions on how to ensure that people who are not fluent in English or those confronted with misinformation can access good information from reliable sources. Ponder replied that a lesson from the REFOCUS project was that ethnicity-specific media platforms are trusted sources of information, and many of those outlets work in the preferred language of marginalized groups. During the COVID-19 pandemic, those platforms were particularly effective at contextualizing health issues and larger issues around the societal, environmental, mental health, and financial effect of the pandemic.

Hunter suggested focusing on the system perspective rather than the consumer perspective. She suggested considering the legal obligations of the health department and other health care organizations to provide information in the languages spoken commonly in the community. She added that a proactive approach to hiring translators and interpreters and issuing communications that are accessible to the community is also important, as well as efforts to help people understand what reliable information is.

The next question asked the panelists to discuss the steps they take when creating health-related messages for target populations. Sharma replied that health care professionals are instructed to avoid using jargon when speaking to patients, but they are not provided instructions on how to do so. This is an area that could be better addressed during provider education and training. She added that speaking to nontechnical people requires talking with humanity, kindness, and grace, not by shaming them, and Sharma mentioned a YouTube channel from Grapevine Health as a place where academics and clinicians can find some lessons for communicating with people outside of their silos.

Ponder recommended the *Pink Book*[2] from the Centers for Disease Control and Prevention and the National Institutes of Health as a tangible source of advice. The *Pink Book* is a colloquial name for a long-standing, trusted resource that includes a step-by-step cycle for how to design a health communication program (National Cancer Institute, 2004). She noted that people in the targeted community will provide insights into what they need to hear and how they need to hear it. Hunter added that her organization's Becoming Better Messengers training, based on Moral Foundations Theory and developed

---

[2] See https://www.cancer.gov/publications/health-communication/pink-book.pdf (accessed September 15, 2022).

based on further research by Burris et al. (2019), starts with understanding the values with which people resonate and the target audience's beliefs and practices, because effective messaging should reflect what people value and what they want to hear (Haidt, 2012). Another good starting point, she added, is to focus on helping people understand how they can engage in a desired activity or take in information.

Considering Community Communicators

Jen Brown asked the panelists to speak about the role of community media and how AHRQ could support researchers to engage with community media. Ponder recommended connecting with journalism advocacy groups such as the National Association of Black Journalists and the National Association of Hispanic Journalists for help making connections to community media. The local health department can be a good source for identifying the important communicators in a community. She also noted that there are many citizen journalists and scientists who are trusted within social spaces and within their community. Those individuals have invested in developing reputations in their community for being a reliable resource of information. It is important as well not to stigmatize or ignore people who may not be "traditional" journalists and work in the digital space but who represent particular communities. In the mass media, there are journalists—for example, science writers or members of the Association of Health Care Journalists—who cover subjects in a culturally and ethnically sound manner and who can write about technical subjects in lay language.

Nikolajski asked the panel to discuss strategies for engaging with community leaders to serve as trusted messengers. Sharma explained that this requires building relationships with those trusted community members and learning how best to engage their expertise. Hunter added that relationships with leaders in the community should be developed proactively. Additionally, health researchers should seek to provide those community leaders with tools and the support to lead conversations instead of leading every conversation themselves. Ponder agreed with Hunter and added that this is an effective approach for empowering community leaders and communities. She added that effective engagement with community leaders requires active listening.

Considering Metrics

The group was next asked to discuss metrics or outcomes for assessing the success of a health communication or health policy initiative or campaign. Hunter said the legal epidemiology framework can be useful for determining how laws affect population and for identifying how specific components of a law affect different health outcomes (Burris et al., 2016; Ramanathan et al., 2017). Sharma said that researchers should be thoughtful about the community they will be engaging and avoid trying to fit all demographics and geographies into one measure. Ponder added that community input is also important when developing measures and suggested using more nontraditional and less quantitative metrics to supplement and complement ongoing work.

Hunter explained that organizations working in a state that has performance-based budgeting are often required to report on measures that are negotiated with legislative analysts and a committee and that may not represent information that is useful for the community. This can result in reporting on a measure for the purpose of meeting a requirement rather than for determining whether a communication effort was effective. She also noted the importance of supporting and engaging the workforce to support the design of measures that do not interfere with workflow.

Considering Levels in the Social Ecologic Framework

Nikolajski asked Ponder to comment on whether there are particular levels in the social ecological framework she discussed that AHRQ should focus on in its health communication strategies. Ponder replied that this varies depending on the goals of a project. In some cases, the work may be most meaningful and effective at the clinician and patient level. In that case communication strategies should focus on collaborating with health care advocacy groups while also ensuring that the work strengthens relationships and provides educational supports. She noted that some issues may be structural, which may involve a different approach that requires more partner-to-partner and institution-to-institution engagement and investigating opportunities to engage policy levels. In instances of public resistance to a message, efforts should be directed at the interpersonal and community levels. One useful exercise is for a team to consider each level in the public health pyramid to develop their communication strategies.

Sharma added that the levels can change, and she would like to see agencies such as AHRQ start investing from the ground up rather than funding big institutions all the time. There are many physicians and nurses, she said, and people with lived experiences who are dynamic communicators and are relatable, reliable, and trusted messengers that are communicating through social media but who are not at a big academic or governmental institution. Hunter noted that local, state, and federal health agencies often have multiple levels of approval for communications. She encouraged research funders to consider how to design flexibility into their communication systems. She noted that during the COVID-19 pandemic, there have been instances of public health departments funding community media partners to establish a more flexible system for communicating with the community.

Engaging Technology

Nikolajski next asked the group to address strategies and opportunities for using technology to effectively communicate public health or public policy information to diverse audiences. Sharma replied that the academic and research community would benefit from increased engagement with digital media platforms. She noted that usually professionals in medicine or science are viewed as experts based on the frequency and quality of their work that is published in scientific journals. However, in order to improve communication of health care research findings, these professionals should also be expected to develop skills in communicating their findings in other settings, such as radio, television, or social media. Ponder remarked that digital tools are an important partner for ensuring information is accessible. This requires researchers to engage in thoughtful communication strategies to ensure information is shared via accessible sources.

Hunter noted that social medial can be a useful tool for communicating health information as well as health care policy related information. She suggested that in order to ensure that accurate information is disseminated, those with expertise should have a presence on social media. She said that these experts have a role in helping people understand the implications of law and policy decisions related to health care for their community.

Training Future Professionals

An unidentified audience member asked the speakers to discuss strategies for integrating these lessons into the education and training of health care professionals and patient-centered outcomes researchers. Sharma suggested that those lessons should be integrated into academic training and incorporated throughout the education process instead of isolated in a single course. Ponder agreed that health communication skills should be incorporated into the academic preparation of all health care and PCOR professionals. She also suggested that researchers could improve the effectiveness of their communication plan by engaging with a health communications professional during the early phases of development of an intervention. She noted that communication training in a project should be considered a structural investment that will generate long-term benefits.

Hunter suggested creating a legal infrastructure to support or require training. She explained that possible approaches to create such a policy include establishing licensure requirements and perhaps a community advisory board with specified duties and responsibilities codified in a legal or policy mechanism that also includes funding. Sharma added that it is important for licensing boards to hold professionals accountable for providing accurate information and not contributing to misinformation or disinformation. Hunter noted that institutional practices should incorporate professional codes of ethics.

Final Thoughts from Speakers

As a final question, Hughes asked the panelists for one message they would give to AHRQ about communications. Ponder said that given that AHRQ's work has broad impact, it would be beneficial for the organization to consider the motivations and implications of their work at all levels of the health care system as well as the communities in which their work is being done. Hunter replied that intervention teams should be intentional in their approach to disseminate information in the community setting as well as the partner engagement piece of their project, whether that is with health care professionals, researchers, or community members. She emphasized the importance of developing processes that facilitate bidirectional conversations with stakeholders to gain feedback regarding existing projects and identify future research priorities. Sharma emphasized the need to seek diverse leaders, which may require considering experts outside their professional networks.

12

Workshop 4, Session 2: Informing Evidence-Based Policy Making

> **Key Messages Presented by Individual Speakers**
> - Researchers should engage with policy stakeholders early in the process of formulating research questions to understand what stakeholders want to know, what time frame is ideal, and what aspects of the research questions have the greatest potential to impact policy. (Tipirneni)
> - Researchers should read the policy or piece of legislation prior to generating research questions to address that legislation or policy. (Tipirneni)
> - Include qualitative research and mixed methods approaches as a powerful way of sharing patient and community perspectives with the health policy community and decision-makers and to understand the outcomes and solutions that patients find important. (Cervantes)
> - Formative audience research can inform effective design of dissemination materials and the channels and sources through which to distribute them. (Purtle)

CONCEPTUALIZING AND CONDUCTING POLICY-RELEVANT RESEARCH

Renuka Tipirneni is an assistant professor in the Department of Internal Medicine and faculty adviser to the policy engagement team at the University of Michigan's Institute for Healthcare Policy and Innovation. She began her presentation by discussing how to pose research questions that will be relevant to health policy. Tipirneni offered suggestions for how to best conceptualize policy-relevant research:

- Read the actual bill, regulation, or court case, for it is essential to understand the details through all the technical language.
- Think of questions that are both interesting and addressable in a time frame that would be useful for policy makers.
- Engage with policy stakeholders early in the process of formulating research questions to understand what those stakeholders want to know, what time frame is ideal, and what aspects of the research questions have the greatest potential to impact policy.

She used her own work evaluating Michigan's Medicaid expansion as an example. When the bill authorizing the state's Medicaid expansion passed, she read each provision of the law and asked herself about the importance of that provision and how she might be able to assess its impact. She paid particular attention to the provision that required the Department of Health to ensure that all Medicaid enrollees have access to primary care and that the department should require all new enrollees to be assigned to and have an appointment scheduled with a primary care physician within 60 days of enrollment, a provision that was later extended to 90 days. Tipirneni noted that as a primary care provider herself, she wondered how the department would be able to ensure and monitor access to primary care providers for patients with Medicaid within those time frames.

Tipirneni considered several methods when she was developing a rigorous study to answer a policy-relevant question that examined both appointment availability and wait times for patients who had Medicaid coverage:

- Conduct a secondary data analysis using federal or state surveys that monitor access to appointments or access to primary care practitioners.
- Analyze visits documented in health care claims data to see when and how often people visited their primary care provider.
- Survey primary care practitioners or their health systems to identify how they are handling capacity issues and if they could meet the demand for patients who needed an appointment within the designated time frame.

- Survey or interview enrollees to ask them whether they were able to get an appointment in a timely manner and if they were able to get the care they needed.
- Conduct a simulated patient, or "secret shopper," study of calling clinics as if one were a patient to see what kind of appointment access was available.

Tipirneni explained that as a member of the formal evaluation team for Michigan's Medicaid expansion, she has used each of these methods for different studies. She said she used the simulated patient method for this particular study because she was interested in both appointment availability and wait times.

Tipirneni offered several suggestions for conducting effective policy-relevant research. She said researchers should first consider a variety of methods, such as secondary data analysis or primary data collection, given that there is no one best approach for considering a research question. Considerations such as time frame for the study, cost, or availability of data should inform method selection. She reiterated that researchers should be cognizant of the allotted time frame when selecting their research method. For example, she ultimately chose to use the simulated patient approach because she needed answers quickly and that was feasible for her and her team. Researchers should incorporate input from collaborating stakeholders when developing and refining the study protocol. She also noted the importance of building a research team that has the necessary expertise and can be nimble to address questions in real time.

Tipirneni next discussed translating research findings to achieve policy impact. She said this process begins with developing products that are useful for different audiences. As an example, she said her team presented the results of a single study in three different forms. She and her collaborators published a traditional peer-reviewed academic paper in a well-respected journal to present results to researchers. The team created an issue brief that it could pair with the journal article for a national audience of both media and policy makers. For stakeholders in the state's Medicaid program—the audience she most wanted to inform—the team prepared an issue brief that she updated regularly as the team collected additional data. The issue brief focused on the information stakeholders prioritized: appointment availability and the regions in the state that had better access and worse access. Tipirneni noted that each document presented the results in a different order and with a different emphasis designed to provide information in a form most accessible and useful for each document's intended audience. The issue briefs, for example, had policy considerations and implications at the start of the document.

Tipirneni offered several overall suggestions for effectively translating research for policy impact, including the following:

- Identifying the target audience and when to disseminate information to the intended audience, including at the local, state, or national level.
- Engaging policy stakeholders early and often.
- Knowing what information the intended audiences are most interested in learning, and present that information in a format that they are accustomed to seeing.
- Writing issue briefs carefully and in a nonpartisan manner, paying close attention to wording so as to not alienate policy makers of one political party.
- Continuing to engage and develop relationships among stakeholders in the research and policy communities to facilitate long term impact.

In closing, Tipirneni summarized her suggestions for researchers seeking to use their study findings to inform policy. Those suggestions included

- reading the policy or piece of legislation prior to generating research questions to address that legislation or policy;
- engaging with policy stakeholders early and often during the research process;
- considering a variety of methods, including secondary data analysis and primary data collection;
- framing research as an iterative process that involves developing questions and methods in collaboration with both researchers and policy stakeholders;
- writing issue briefs, not just academic papers, to translate research findings for policy stakeholders; and
- developing relationships with policy makers and maintain them over time to truly have an impact on policy.

CHANGING ACCESS TO CARE FOR UNDOCUMENTED IMMIGRANTS WITH DATA

Lilia Cervantes is director of immigrant health and an associate professor in the Department of Medicine at the University of Colorado Anschutz Medical Campus. She began by describing the Latina/o community in the United States. They are a heterogeneous population with respect to immigration generation and status, country, language of origin, and race. She said the Latino community faces a disproportionate burden of social challenges. She said the poverty rate among Latinos is 17 percent, about double the poverty rate among non-Latino White individuals. In addition, nearly a third of individuals in the Latino community report limited English proficiency, and Latino patients often do not have access to interpreters when needed in health care systems. She said the 8 million members of the Latino community that are undocumented are the least likely of any racial or ethnic group to have health insurance.

Cervantes explained that she was inspired to pursue research as a means of changing health policy when caring for a patient with end-stage kidney disease who was undocumented and a mother of two boys. Instead of receiving dialysis three times a week, she came to the hospital every 7 days for emergency dialysis when she was critically ill. Her two sons faced significant physical and psychosocial distress on a weekly basis because they did not know if their mother would survive to the following week. After her third cardiac arrest, the patient decided to stop emergency dialysis, found a couple to adopt her sons, and passed away on Mother's Day 2014.

Cervantes explained that U.S. citizens can receive Medicare-covered kidney replacement therapy, including dialysis and kidney transplantation, because of the 1972 Medicare end-stage renal disease entitlement program.[1] However, the availability of kidney replacement therapy varies by state for undocumented immigrants, who are excluded from Medicare, most Medicaid programs, and provisions of the Affordable Care Act. In 1986, Congress passed the Emergency Medical Treatment and Active Labor Act,[2] which prohibits refusal of care in an emergency situation regardless of immigration or insurance status. Cervantes said this legislation motivated every state to create its own emergency Medicaid program. Many states adopted the Emergency Medical Treatment and Active Labor Act's exact language that only requires reimbursement for care when an undocumented immigrant is critically ill. She explained that the Centers for Medicare and Medicaid Services (CMS) does not provide regulatory guidance defining an emergency medical condition, instead deferring to the states to determine the qualifying conditions (Figure 12-1).

While considering how to change policy in her state of Colorado, Cervantes found a perspective article that challenged the nephrology community, and physicians in general, to obtain more data to best define options to reform state policies for undocumented immigrants with kidney failure (Straube, 2009). She began by engaging various stakeholders in qualitative research and connecting with decision makers to identify the research questions that they felt were important and whose answers could persuade them to change policy. Patients were her primary partners in this work, so she also

---

[1] *Social Security Amendment of 1972*, Public Law 603, 92nd Cong., 1st sess. (October 30, 1972) §2991.

[2] *Emergency Medical Treatment and Active Labor Act*, 41 U.S.C. § 1395dd.

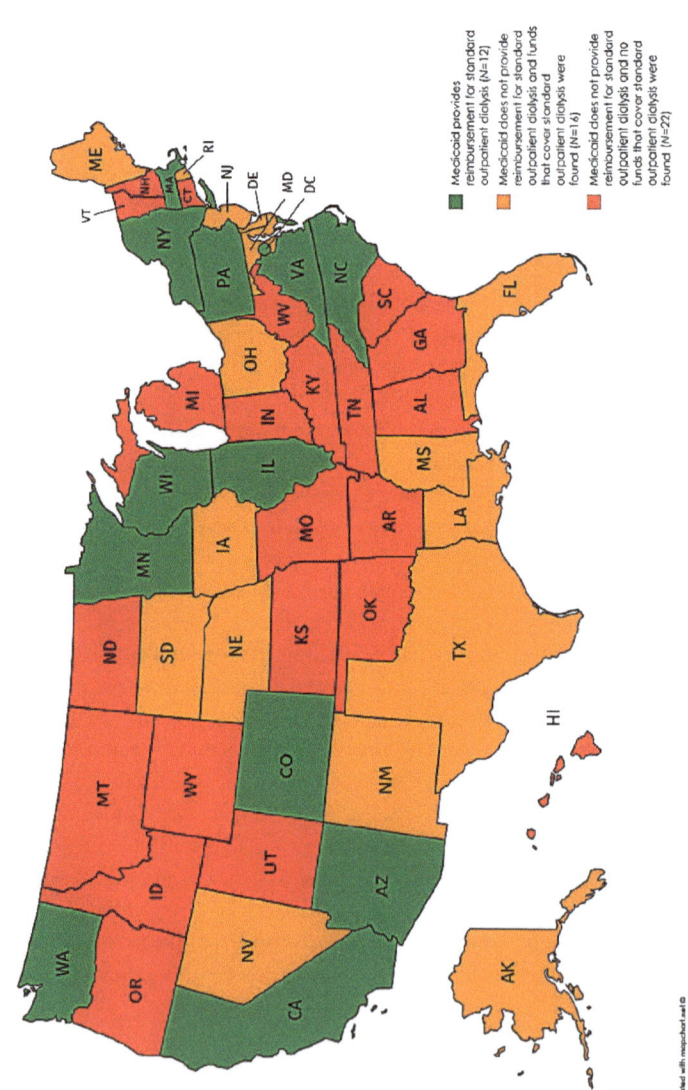

FIGURE 12-1 Medicaid-covered provision of standard dialysis for undocumented immigrants in 2019
SOURCE: Used with permission of the American Society of Nephrology, from The Status of Provision of Standard Outpatient Dialysis for US Undocumented Immigrants with ESKD, Vol. 14 Issue 8, 2017; permission conveyed through Copyright Clearance Center, Inc. Presented by Lilia Cervantes on July 6, 2022, at Accelerating the Use of Findings from Patient-Centered Outcomes Research in Clinical Practice to Improve Health and Health Care: A Workshop Series (Cervantes et al., 2019).

conducted qualitative interviews with patients and their families (Cervantes et al., 2020a). She and her colleagues also conducted qualitative interviews with 50 interdisciplinary clinicians and learned that many of them faced burnout from witnessing needless suffering and high mortality, experienced physical exhaustion from overextending themselves to provide bridge care, and were detaching so as to numb themselves from feeling too much empathy for these patients (Cervantes et al., 2018a).

Cervantes also assessed mortality change or mortality differences between patients who rely on emergency dialysis and those that receive standard dialysis. The results showed that patients who receive emergency dialysis had a 14-fold greater mortality within 5 years of initiating dialysis and a nearly 10-fold greater utilization of services resulting from emergency department visits and hospitalization (Cervantes et al., 2018b). She said that at the time of her study, investigators in Dallas, Texas, were conducting a study in which they enrolled a subset of undocumented immigrants with kidney failure into private health insurance off the state insurance exchange thanks to a private philanthropist (Nguyen et al., 2019). The research team followed the patients for a year and assessed mortality and cost. They found patients who received emergency dialysis had a mortality that was five-fold greater at 1 year than patients enrolled in private insurance who were able to receive standard care (Nguyen et al., 2019). In addition, care for patients who went on standard dialysis cost approximately $6,000 per person per month less than the cost of care for those who relied on emergency dialysis.

Cervantes and her collaborators developed relationships with community-based organizations while conducting their research. Those community-based organizations were able to connect them with policy stakeholders including the state Medicaid agency and the governor's office. Cervantes and her colleagues provided policy stakeholders with research evidence to support policy change. Colorado's Medicaid agency decided in February 2019 to expand access to standard dialysis by including it as a service under the Emergency Medicaid Program.

Cervantes collaborated with a former state Medicaid director and several other colleagues to write a piece for the *Clinical Journal of the American Society of Nephrologists* that described the steps they took to achieve this policy change (Cervantes et al., 2020b). She also partnered with the National Kidney Foundation to send an open letter to state Medicaid directors, co-signed by several national physician organizations, outlining this issue and describing the steps to create policy change (American College of Physicians Colorado Chapter et al., 2021).

Cervantes and her colleagues continue to engage in the evidence dissemination strategies they learned from the dialysis project to address other health care policy matters. During the COVID-19 pandemic, Cervantes and her colleagues learned that patients who were undocumented did not have access to outpatient COVID-19 care. Cervantes and her collaborators conducted a qualitative study that identified several themes: patients described misinformation and disbelief; they relied heavily on social media for information about COVID-19; they thought COVID-19 was a compounder of disadvantage because they had no safeguards such as health insurance or paid sick leave; and they described a reluctance to seek medical care because they worried about being turned away or deported or about the cost of care (Cervantes et al., 2021a). A retrospective analysis of all individuals who had been hospitalized since the onset of the pandemic found that of the 1,000 people she and her collaborators identified, Latinas/os accounted for two-thirds of the hospitalizations and half of the deaths (Podewils et al., 2020). Cervantes and her colleagues combined those qualitative and quantitative research findings to present evidence to support policy change to the state Medicaid agency. This contributed to an expansion of emergency Medicaid care to include outpatient COVID-19 as a qualifying condition. Cervantes and her collaborators used their data to reduce misinformation throughout the state. They also received funding to launch a community health worker program that provided culture- and language-concordant COVID-19 information and COVID-19 vaccinations.

Cervantes closed by noting her team received three times as many media requests to highlight an issue after publishing their qualitative findings compared to when they published their quantitative findings. She said qualitative and mixed methods research can provide needed context when communicating research evidence to policy makers.

DISSEMINATION RESEARCH TO PROMOTE EVIDENCE-INFORMED POLICY MAKING

Jonathan Purtle is an associate professor of public health policy in management and director of policy research at New York University's Global Center for Implementation Science. He began by explaining policy making is more of an art than a science, but he would be addressing the science part of policy making (specifically, dissemination research). He would also discuss how he and his collaborators have applied research methods to determine how to better infuse research evidence into policy making processes. Dissemination research, he explained, is a branch within the broader field of implementation science that is concerned with packaging and communicating research evidence to different audiences. According to the National Institutes of Health definition, "dissemination research is the scientific study of targeted distribution of information and intervention materials to a specific public health or clinical practice audience. The intent of dissemination research is to understand how best to spread and sustain knowledge and the associated evidence-based interventions."[3]

Purtle said he was drawn to the field of dissemination research because he wanted to understand how to translate high-quality, policy-relevant research into public policy in general and state legislation in particular. He said most of the 7,383 state legislators in the United States do not have expertise in health issues. "We want to understand how to shape their knowledge and their attitudes in ways that are aligned with evidence," said Purtle, "and we want the best policies on the books from a population health and health equity perspective." He explained dissemination research resembles communication research in that the goal is to understand how to better communicate about research. However, dissemination research is unique in that dissemination involves communicating about evidence to a clinical practice audience. He noted that the Agency for Healthcare Research and Quality (AHRQ) published a systematic review of communication and dissemination strategies focused mainly on health care providers (McCormack et al., 2013). Purtle and his colleagues published a review in 2020 that laid out a three-phase approach to conducting dissemination research (Purtle et al., 2020).

Purtle said his work, which is focused on policy makers, is informed by a personal observation that while systematic reviews present intensively reviewed evidence for developing practice guidelines, a policy brief is typically based on anecdotal evidence. "We contend that by doing research about the dissemination of research evidence, we can improve how evidence spreads, and we can change knowledge and attitudes in policy makers in ways that we want to see," said Purtle. He added the caveat that while dissemination research can improve how evidence spreads, it does not guarantee that evidence will consistently inform policy because of the nature of the policy making process,

The first phase for dissemination is to conduct formative audience research. He said formative audience research is the broad, descriptive research to understand a target audience of policy makers. This phase informs how to design dissemination materials and the channels and sources through which to distribute them. Purtle explained that the first aim of formative audience research is to gain information about the intended audience's awareness of the problem a given policy is seeking to address. "Often, as researchers, we have deep content expertise and solutions to problems, but state legislators and the general public do not see those problems as problems yet. They do not have the background information so often we have to educate them about that first before we can share evidence about policy solutions," said Purtle. For example, Purtle and his collaborators surveyed 475 U.S. state legislators to see if they

---

[3] Available at https://grants.nih.gov/grants/guide/pa-files/PAR-18-007.html (accessed September 14, 2022).

were aware of the large body of epidemiologic evidence showing that adverse childhood experiences are risk factors for mental health and substance use issues in adolescence and adulthood (Purtle et al., 2019a). Knowing whether their knowledge aligned with the evidence on this particular issue would help inform what a policy brief might emphasize or not need to emphasize. Formative audience research also aims to determine policy makers' attitudes about a specific evidence-supported policy. When Purtle's team surveyed legislators' attitudes related to state behavioral health parity laws, they found that nearly three-quarters of the legislators believed the evidence that parity laws increase access to behavioral health (Purtle et al., 2019b). However, only around half of the legislators believed the evidence that mental health and substance use disorder treatments can be effective, and only 16 percent believed the evidence that parity laws do not increase insurance premiums. These results helped the team identify topics around which to design research. Purtle and his collaborators also found that 40 percent of legislators surveyed did support behavioral health parity laws (Purtle et al., 2019b). The research team also looked at the adjusted odds ratio comparing whether legislators supported such laws and their beliefs about the effectiveness of those laws, the associated costs, treatment effectiveness, and political ideology. The team used that analysis to gain insight into the types of knowledge or attitudes they might want to shift to enhance support for policy aligned with evidence.

The second phase of dissemination research is audience segmentation research. Audience segmentation research seeks to generate data to inform how to design and distribute dissemination materials specifically to different groups of policy makers and legislators within a given target audience. Purtle said conducting audience segmentation research is standard practice in marketing, advertising, and health communications. He explained the general premise of audience segmentation research is that there will be a great deal of heterogeneity in a population in terms of their knowledge, attitudes, and behaviors related to a specific issue. There are two ways to conduct audience segmentation research: demographic separation and empirical clustering. Demographic separation involves stratifying an audience by a demographic variable of interest. For example, liberal, moderate, and conservative legislators have different opinions about the role of adverse childhood experiences as risk factors for adult behavioral health conditions (Table 12-1) (Purtle et al., 2019a). Empirical clustering uses a method such as latent class analysis or K-means clustering to identify different audience segments (Hagenaars and McCutcheon, 2002; Shukla and Naganna, 2014). From the same survey of 475 state legislators, Purtle identified three different audience segments related to the effectiveness of behavioral health and substance use disorder treatments: budget-oriented skeptics with a negative bias toward people with mental illness, passive supporters, and action-oriented supporters (Purtle et al., 2018). The research

TABLE 12-1 Audience Segmentation According to Beliefs About Mental Health and Substance Use Disorder

	Budget-Oriented Skeptics with Stigma (47%)	Action-Oriented Supporters (24%)	Passive Supporters (29%)
Strong agreement that mental health treatments can help people with mental illness lead normal lives	16.9%	73.8%	98.9%
Strong agreement that substance disorder treatments can help people with a substance use disorder recovers	12.6%	78.5%	84.8%
1st quartile (least stigma)	12.0%	47.1%	46.6%
2nd quartile	11.2%	19.6%	27.1%
3rd quartile	42.6%	23.2%	18.5%
4th quartile (most stigma)	34.2%	10.1%	7.8%
Extent to which the bill is going to impact the state budget	51.4%	29.2%	40.5%
Extent to which the bill is based on scientific evidence	46.1%	74.1%	72.7%
Mental health	29.3%	45.0%	43.0%
Substance use	41.1%	58.3%	40.2%
Mental health	13.4%	90.7%	23.2%
Substance use	15.4%	96.3%	4.6%

SOURCE: https://implementationscience.biomedcentral.com/articles/10.1186/s13012-018-0816-8. Used under Creative Commons license CC BY 4.0, available at https://creativecommons.org/licenses/by/4.0/. No changes made. Presented by Jonathan Purtle on July 6, 2022, at Accelerating the Use of Findings from Patient-Centered Outcomes Research in Clinical Practice to Improve Health and Health Care: A Workshop Series (data from Purtle et al., 2019a).

team then input different variables into the latent class analysis for these three groups to identify factors that would influence their support for a behavioral health bill that would be introduced in their state legislature. Purtle explained that based on the results of that analysis, "we can think about how we might craft a policy brief and messages for legislators in the budget-oriented skeptics with stigma [negative bias] group that might be much different from what we emphasize in a policy brief and messages for legislators in the action-oriented supporter or passive supporter groups."

The third phase of dissemination research focused on policy makers is dissemination effectiveness research. Dissemination effectiveness research involves conducting randomized controlled trials of different dissemination strategies to see which strategies are most effective. As an example, Purtle discussed a cluster-randomized controlled trial of all U.S. state legislatures to determine how much it matters to legislators if dissemination materials include economic evidence and how much it matters to have state-tailored evidence as opposed to national data (Purtle et al., 2022). His team randomized states and disseminated different policy briefs by email. The research team then tracked engagement with the evidence by email views and the rate at which legislators clicked links in the email to view the policy briefs. All the emails concluded with an offer for expert consultation for more information, which they tracked as an outcome. They also tracked mentions of adverse childhood experiences and related terms on legislators' social media accounts two months after sending materials. The results, said Purtle, indicated that including economic evidence increased engagement with dissemination materials among Democrats but not Republicans, which they did not expect (Purtle et al., 2022). He said that finding was useful when crafting different dissemination plans to reach Democrats and Republicans.

Purtle concluded his remarks with a quote from the late scholar Carol H. Weiss, who said, "The policy making process is a political process, with the basic aim of reconciling interests in order to negotiate a consensus, not of implementing logic and truth. The value issues in policy making cannot be settled by referring to research findings." Purtle said policy making is a political act, something researchers such as himself find frustrating, but it is an important reality to embrace because it is not going to change.

DISCUSSION

Strengthening Relationships between Researchers and Policy Makers

Session moderator Lauren Hughes opened the discussion by asking the panelists for insights on how to strengthen the relationships between policy makers and researchers. Cervantes replied that she had success with using the connections she had with community-based organizations who had relationships with policy makers. Purtle suggested identifying the legislators who have a demonstrated interest in an issue to be addressed and reaching out to them specifically to start cultivating a relationship. He noted researchers should consider reaching out as constituents to their own elective officials.

Considerations for Informing Policy

Hughes asked the panelists to discuss how to effectively leverage narrative evidence to advance policy. Cervantes suggested researchers engage patients and stakeholders who are interested in the issue to be addressed. Researchers can use stories from those patients and stakeholders as narrative evidence to present to a legislator or decision maker as an illustration of what patients and stakeholders want to be part of a solution to the issue. She includes quotes from patients and stakeholders in policy briefs and brings patients and other stakeholders to meetings. Purtle added that narratives work to influence policy makers because, as research has shown, they are more engaging and easier to process than experimental results and data. However, narratives can have unintended consequences. He cited one study showing that narratives work to garner support from Democrats for policies that would improve food security, but that they reduced support among Republicans.

Hughes asked speakers to discuss approaches for conceptualizing policy-relevant questions, Purtle replied that he seeks as many perspectives as possible. Cervantes agreed with Purtle, and noted the importance of including opponents to the policy to be addressed to get their perspectives. She also finds understanding the policy pathway in other states and the data that produced change in those states to be informative.

Considering Different Dissemination Tools

Hughes asked the panelists for examples of dissemination products beyond peer-reviewed publications that they have found useful in their work. Cervantes said she found social medal useful, adding that a Twitter tutorial comprising a series of tweets, each with a specific nugget of information, proved important in both her kidney dialysis and COVID-19 projects. She also noted the importance of including patients in dissemination efforts because they are often unaware of policies that can benefit them. Purtle agreed that Twitter is a useful dissemination tool, especially if the tweet contains links to additional information so that users can click and learn more about an issue. He also includes his phone number in emails and policy briefs that he sends to legislators, which often results in phone calls from the legislator or staff member.

Supporting Translating Research to Policy

An audience member then asked speakers to discuss their ideas for how AHRQ or other funders can support infrastructure development at research institutions and provide incentives to support researchers who want to engage in the policy space. Purtle noted that many academics are hesitant to work on policy issues because they believe they will be penalized in terms of tenure and promotion, so perhaps AHRQ could emphasize that this type of work should be valued, rewarded, and supported. Cervantes added that academic institutions are realizing that service and engagement in advocacy work is important for promotion. In that regard, AHRQ funding mechanisms could shift some of its funding to reflect policy change as an important endpoint for research, particularly as it affects upstream drivers of health inequities. She suggested AHRQ might also develop a curriculum that would educate clinicians and researchers about engaging in research that changes policy. She said such a curriculum would include how to put a policy brief together and how to think about research questions that can lead to policy change.

Speakers' Advice for Researchers

Hughes asked the panelists what advice they would give to a colleague considering engaging in policy-related work. Cervantes said that she advises her medical students and residents who want to engage in policy that it is important to engage with stakeholders, particularly community-based organizations, who have policy experience and can lend their expertise. Purtle noted that to a newcomer, policy making can seem so complex that it is overwhelming. He advises people interested in engaging in policy work to first identify the exact policy that needs changing, who has the authority to change that policy, and narrow the issue to a reasonable scale.

CLOSING SUMMARY OF WORKSHOP 4

Hughes concluded the workshop by summarizing her takeaways from the presentations and discussions. She described several key points highlighted by speakers about various aspects of effective communication of research findings:[4]

- Being aware of the effect of language on how the message is conveyed and its reach
- Engaging trusted messengers who look and sound like the patients and families that research is intending to serve
- Remembering the public, separate from patients, providers, and policy makers, is a critical constituency to which dissemination of information needs to occur

---

[4] These points were made by the individual workshop speakers/participants identified above. They are not intended to reflect a consensus among workshop participants.

- Communicating research findings to the public, patients, providers, and policy makers frequently requires the message to get through a great deal of noise, stress, and inequities in the current system
- Considering the effects of health literacy and readiness to change when planning communication efforts
- Understanding how subject matter experts can use media platforms to disseminate accurate information
- Considering integrating health communications professionals into a research team to support effective dissemination

Hughes noted that speakers provided several suggestions to guide researchers to develop policy-relevant research questions including: reading the bill, law, or court case to be addressed by the research and determining whether the research question is realistic and addressable within a specified time frame. Hughes noted there was a substantial discussion about translating evidence into policy and approaches for disseminating research findings to policy makers that goes beyond authoring peer-reviewed papers for the academic literature. Speakers had several suggestions for best approaches to disseminating research evidence to policy makers including[5]

- Knowing the audience, including those who hold different opinions
- Selecting communication materials that are most effective and useful for each audience
- Avoiding language that could alienate policy makers of one political party
- Incorporating narrative evidence to provide context to quantitative data
- Understanding the baseline awareness of the evidence and attitudes toward interventions among policy makers
- Conducting audience segmentation to better understand knowledge, attitudes, and behaviors that will inform and allow for tailoring communications and dissemination plans

---

[5] These points were made by the individual workshop speakers/participants identified above. They are not intended to reflect a consensus among workshop participants.

References

Abernethy, A., L. Adams, M. Barrett, C. Bechtel, P. Brennan, A. Butte, J. Faulkner, E. Fontaine, S. Friedhoff, J. Halamka, M. Howell, K. Johnson, P. Lee, P. Long, D. McGraw, R. Miller, J. Perlin, D. Rucker, L. Sandy, L. Savage, L. Stump, P. Tang, E. Topol, R. Tuckson, and K. Valdes. 2022. *The promise of digital health: Then, now, and the future.* Washington, DC: National Academy of Medicine.

Adams, L., S. Kennedy, L. Allen, A. Barnes, T. Bias, D. Crane, P. Lanier, R. Mauk, S. Mohamoud, N. Pauly, J. Talbert, C. Woodcock, K. Zivin, and J. Donohue. 2019. Innovative solutions for state Medicaid programs to leverage their data, build their analytic capacity, and create evidence-based policy. *EGEMS (Washington, DC)* 7(1):41.

Afzal, M., N. Siddiqi, B. Ahmad, N. Afsheen, F. Aslam, A. Ali, R. Ayesha, M. Bryant, R. Holt, H. Khalid, K. Ishaq, K. N. Koly, S. Rajan, J. Saba, N. Tirbhowan, and G. A. Zavala. 2021. Prevalence of overweight and obesity in people with severe mental illness: Systematic review and meta-analysis. *Frontiers in Endocrinology (Lausanne)* 12:769309.

AHRQ (Agency for Healthcare Research and Quality). 2016. *Potential of the Patient-Centered Outcomes Research Trust Fund.* https://www.ahrq.gov/pcor/potential-of-the-pcortf/index.html (accessed September 14, 2022).

AHRQ. 2022. *AHRQ's patient-centered outcomes research strategic framework.* https://www.ahrq.gov/pcor/strategic-framework/index.html (accessed Septernber 15, 2022).

American College of Physicians Colorado Chapter, American Society of Nephrology, American Thoracic Society, Endocrine Society, Home Dialyzors United, Kidney Care Partners, National Kidney Foundation, Renal Physicians Association, Society of General Internal Medicine, and Society of Hospital Medicine. 2021. *Open letter to state Medicaid directors*. New York, NY: National Kidney Foundation.

Ananth, C. V., K. M. Keyes, and R. J. Wapner. 2013. Pre-eclampsia rates in the United States, 1980-2010: Age-period-cohort analysis. *BMJ: British Medical Journal* 347:f6564.

APHA (American Public Health Association). 2022. *Community Health Workers*. https://www.apha.org/apha-communities/member-sections/community-health-workers (accessed September 15, 2022).

Askie, L. M., L. Duley, D. J. Henderson-Smart, and L. A. Stewart. 2007. Antiplatelet agents for prevention of pre-eclampsia: A meta-analysis of individual patient data. *Lancet* 369(9575):1791-1798.

Bailey, Z. D., N. Krieger, M. Agénor, J. Graves, N. Linos, and M. T. Bassett. 2017. Structural racism and health inequities in the USA: Evidence and interventions. *Lancet* 389(10077):1453-1463.

Baron, R. M., and D. A. Kenny. 1986. The moderator-mediator variable distinction in social psychological research: Conceptual, strategic, and statistical considerations. *Journal of Personality and Social Psychology* 51(6):1173-1182.

Bauer, M. S., L. Damschroder, H. Hagedorn, J. Smith, and A. M. Kilbourne. 2015. An introduction to implementation science for the non-specialist. *BMC Psychology* 3(1):32. doi: 10.1186/s40359-015-0089-9.

Baumann, A., M. Domenech Rodríguez, and J. R. Parra-Cardona. 2011. Community-based applied research with Latino immigrant families: Informing practice and research according to ethical and social justice principles. *Family Process* 50(2):132-148.

Baumann, A. A., and L. J. Cabassa. 2020. Reframing implementation science to address inequities in healthcare delivery. *BMC Health Services Research* 20(1):190.

Baumann, A. A., and P. D. Long. 2021. Equity in implementation science is long overdue. *Stanford Social Innovation Review* 19(3):A15-A17.

Branham, D. K., K. Finegold, L. Chen, M. Sorbero, R. Euller, M. N. Elliott, and B. D. Sommers. 2022. Trends in missing race and ethnicity information after imputation in healthcare.gov marketplace enrollment data, 2015-2021. *JAMA Network Open* 5(6):e2216715.

Brooks, D., M. Douglas, N. Aggarwal, S. Prabhakaran, K. Holden, and D. Mack. 2017. Developing a framework for integrating health equity into the learning health system. *Learning Health Systems* 1(3):e10029.

Brownson, R. C., J. E. Fielding, and C. M. Maylahn. 2009. Evidence-based public health: A fundamental concept for public health practice. *Annual Review of Public Health* 30:175-201.

Brownson, R. C., R. C. Shelton, E. H. Geng, and R. E. Glasgow. 2022. Revisiting concepts of evidence in implementation science. *Implementation Science* 17(1):26.

Burris, S., M. Ashe, D. Levin, M. Penn, and M. Larkin. 2016. A transdisciplinary approach to public health law: The emerging practice of legal epidemiology. *Annual Review of Public Health* 37(1):135-148.

Burris, S., G. Matthews, G. Gunderson, and E. L. Baker. 2019. Becoming better messengers: The public health advantage. *Journal of Public Health Management and Practice* 25(4).

CDC (Centers for Disease Control and Prevention). 2022. Community Health Worker (CHW) Toolkit. https://www.cdc.gov/dhdsp/pubs/toolkits/chw-toolkit.htm (accessed September 14, 2022).

Cervantes, L., S. Richardson, R. Raghavan, N. Hou, R. Hasnain-Wynia, M. K. Wynia, C. Kleiner, M. Chonchol, and A. Tong. 2018a. Clinicians' perspectives on providing emergency-only hemodialysis to undocumented immigrants: A qualitative study. *Annals of Internal Medicine* 169(2):78-86.

Cervantes, L., D. Tuot, R. Raghavan, S. Linas, J. Zoucha, L. Sweeney, C. Vangala, M. Hull, M. Camacho, A. Keniston, C. E. McCulloch, V. Grubbs, J. Kendrick, and N. R. Powe. 2018b. Association of emergency-only vs standard hemodialysis with mortality and health care use among undocumented immigrants with end-stage renal disease. *JAMA Internal Medicine* 178(2):188-195.

Cervantes, L., W. Mundo, and N. R. Powe. 2019. The status of provision of standard outpatient dialysis for US undocumented immigrants with ESKD. *Clinical Journal of the American Society of Nephrology* 14(8):1258.

Cervantes, L., A. L. Carr, C. C. Welles, J. Zoucha, J. F. Steiner, T. Johnson, M. Earnest, C. Camacho, K. Suresh, and R. Hasnain-Wynia. 2020a. The experience of primary caregivers of undocumented immigrants with end-stage kidney disease that rely on emergency-only hemodialysis. *Journal of General Internal Medicine* 35(8):2389-2397.

Cervantes, L., T. Johnson, A. Hill, and M. Earnest. 2020b. Offering better standards of dialysis care for immigrants: The Colorado example. *Clinical Journal of the American Society of Nephrology* 15(10):1516-1518.

Cervantes, L., M. Martin, M. G. Frank, J. F. Farfan, M. Kearns, L. A. Rubio, A. Tong, A. Matus Gonzalez, C. Camacho, A. Collings, W. Mundo, N. R. Powe, and A. Fernandez. 2021. Experiences of Latinx individuals hospitalized for COVID-19: A qualitative study. *JAMA Network Open* 4(3):e210684.

CIBHS (California Institute for Behavioral Health Solutions). 2015. *What is a Learning Collaborative?* https://work.cibhs.org/overview/whatlearning-collaborative (accessed September 14, 2022).

Davidson, K. W., S. Ye, and G. A. Mensah. 2017. Commentary: De-implementation science: A virtuous cycle of ceasing and desisting low-value care before implementing new high value care. *Ethnicity & Disease* 27(4):463.

De Hert, M., J. M. Dekker, D. Wood, K. G. Kahl, R. I. Holt, and H. J. Möller. 2009. Cardiovascular disease and diabetes in people with severe mental illness: Position statement from the European Psychiatric Association (EPA), supported by the European Association for the Study of Diabetes (EASD) and the European Society of Cardiology (ESC). *European Psychiatry* 24(6):412-424.

Dearing, J. W., and J. G. Cox. 2018. Diffusion of innovations theory, principles, and practice. *Health Affairs* 37(2):183-190.

Delgado, M. K., A. U. Morgan, D. A. Asch, R. Xiong, A. S. Kilaru, K. C. Lee, D. Do, A. B. Friedman, Z. F. Meisel, C. K. Snider, D. Lam, A. Parambath, C. Wood, C. M. Wilson, M. Perez, D. L. Chisholm, S. Kelly, C. J. O'Malley, N. Mannion, A. M. Huffenberger, S. McGinley, M. Balachandran, N. Khan, N. Mitra, and K. H. Chaiyachati. 2021. Comparative effectiveness of an automated text messaging service for monitoring COVID-19 at home. *Annals of Internal Medicine* 175(2):179-190.

Donohue, J., A. C. Raslevich, and E. Cole. 2022. *Medicaid's role in improving substance use disorder in the US.* New York, NY: Milbank Memorial Fund.

Eccles, M. P., and B. S. Mittman. 2006. Welcome to implementation science. *Implementation Science* 1(1):1.

Escoffery, C., K. Glanz, and T. Elliott. 2008. Process evaluation of the Pool Cool diffusion trial for skin cancer prevention across 2 years. *Health Education Research* 23(4):732-743.

Farhang, L., and X. Morales. 2022. *Building community power to achieve health and racial equity: Principles to guide transformative partnerships with local communities.* Washington, DC: National Academy of Medicine.

Frieden, T. R. 2010. A framework for public health action: The health impact pyramid. *American Journal of Public Health* 100(4):590-595.

Gaglio, B., J. A. Shoup, and R. E. Glasgow. 2013. The RE-AIM framework: A systematic review of use over time. *American Journal of Public Health* 103(6):e38-e46.

Ghulmiyyah, L., and B. Sibai. 2012. Maternal mortality from preeclampsia/eclampsia. *Seminars in Perinatology* 36(1):56-59.

Gies, P., K. Glanz, D. O'Riordan, T. Elliott, and E. Nehl. 2009. Measured occupational solar UVR exposures of lifeguards in pool settings. *American Journal of Industrial Medicine* 52(8):645-653.

Glanz, K., F. McCarty, E. J. Nehl, D. L. O'Riordan, P. Gies, L. Bundy, A. E. Locke, and D. M. Hall. 2009. Validity of self-reported sunscreen use by parents, children, and lifeguards. *American Journal of Preventive Medicine* 36(1):63-69.

Glanz, K., P. Gies, D. L. O'Riordan, T. Elliott, E. Nehl, F. McCarty, and E. Davis. 2010. Validity of self-reported solar UVR exposure compared with objectively measured UVR exposure. *Cancer Epidemiology, Biomarkers & Prevention* 19(12):3005-3012.

Glanz, K., C. Escoffery, T. Elliott, and E. J. Nehl. 2015. Randomized trial of two dissemination strategies for a skin cancer prevention program in aquatic settings. *American Journal of Public Health* 105(7):1415-1423.

REFERENCES

Glasgow, R. E., S. M. Harden, B. Gaglio, B. Rabin, M. L. Smith, G. C. Porter, M. G. Ory, and P. A. Estabrooks. 2019. RE-AIM planning and evaluation framework: Adapting to new science and practice with a 20-year review. *Frontiers in Public Health* 7:64.

Göttgens, I., and S. Oertelt-Prigione. 2021. The application of human-centered design approaches in health research and innovation: A narrative review of current practices. *JMIR mHealth and uHealth* 9(12):e28102. doi: 10.2196/28102.

Graham, A. K., J. E. Wildes, M. Reddy, S. A. Munson, C. Barr Taylor, and D. C. Mohr. 2019. User-centered design for technology-enabled services for eating disorders. *International Journal of Eating Disorders* 52(10):1095-1107.

Graham, A. K., C. J. Greene, M. J. Kwasny, S. M. Kaiser, P. Lieponis, T. Powell, and D. C. Mohr. 2020a. Coached mobile app platform for the treatment of depression and anxiety among primary care patients: A randomized clinical trial. *JAMA Psychiatry* 77(9):906-914.

Graham, A. K., C. J. Greene, T. Powell, P. Lieponis, A. Lunsford, C. D. Peralta, L. C. Orr, S. M. Kaiser, N. Alam, H. Berhane, O. Kalan, and D. C. Mohr. 2020b. Lessons learned from service design of a trial of a digital mental health service: Informing implementation in primary care clinics. *Translational Behavioral Medicine* 10(3):598-605.

Graham, A. K., E. G. Lattie, B. J. Powell, A. R. Lyon, J. D. Smith, S. M. Schueller, N. A. Stadnick, C. H. Brown, and D. C. Mohr. 2020c. Implementation strategies for digital mental health interventions in health care settings. *The American Psychologist* 75(8):1080-1092.

Green, L. W., J. M. Ottoson, C. Garcia, and R. A. Hiatt. 2009. Diffusion theory and knowledge dissemination, utilization, and integration in public health. *Annual Review of Public Health* 30:151-174.

Hagenaars, J. A., and A. L. McCutcheon. 2002. *Applied latent class analysis.* Cambridge, UK: Cambridge University Press.

Haidt, J. 2012. *The rightous mind: Why good people are divided by politics and religion.* New York, NY: Vintage Books.

Hall, D., N. Dubruiel, T. Elliott, and K. Glanz. 2009. Linking agents' activities and communication patterns in a study of the dissemination of an effective skin cancer prevention program. *Journal of Public Health Management and Practice* 15(5):409-415.

Holtrop, J. S., B. A. Rabin, and R. E. Glasgow. 2018. Dissemination and implementation science in primary care research and practice: Contributions and opportunities. *The Journal of the American Board of Family Medicine* 31(3):466-478.

Hooker, L., R. Small, C. Humphreys, K. Hegarty, and A. Taft. 2015. Applying normalization process theory to understand implementation of a family violence screening and care model in maternal and child health nursing practice: A mixed method process evaluation of a randomised controlled trial. *Implementation Science* 10:39.

Hooker, L., and A. Taft. 2016. Using theory to design, implement and evaluate sustained nurse domestic violence screening and supportive care. *Journal of Research in Nursing* 21(5-6):432-442.

Institute of Medicine. 1983. *Community oriented primary care: New directions for health services delivery.* Washington, DC: The National Academies Press.

Institute of Medicine. 1984a. *Community oriented primary care: A practical assessment, vol. 1: Report of a study.* Washington, DC: The National Academies Press.

Institute of Medicine. 1984b. *Community oriented primary care: A practical assessment, vol. 2: Case studies.* Washington, DC: The National Academies Press.

Jarlenski, M., J. Y. Kim, K. A. Ahrens, L. Allen, A. Austin, A. J. Barnes, D. Crane, P. Lanier, R. Mauk, S. Mohamoud, N. Pauly, J. Talbert, K. Zivin, and J. M. Donohue. 2021. Healthcare patterns of pregnant women and children affected by OUD in 9 state Medicaid populations. *Journal of Addiction Medicine* 15(5):406-413.

Jemmott, J. B., 3rd, L. S. Jemmott, A. O'Leary, L. D. Icard, S. E. Rutledge, R. Stevens, J. Hsu, and A. J. Stephens. 2015. On the efficacy and mediation of a one-on-one HIV risk-reduction intervention for African American men who have sex with men: A randomized controlled trial. *AIDS and Behavior* 19(7):1247-1262.

Jones, J., and S. Muller. 2018. *Social determinants of health and Medicaid payments.* Madison, WI: Deloitte Center for Government Insights.

Kangovi, S., N. Mitra, D. Grande, J. A. Long, and D. A. Asch. 2020. Evidence-based community health worker program addresses unmet social needs and generates positive return on investment. *Health Affairs (Millwood)* 39(2):207-213.

Kangovi, S., N. Mitra, L. Norton, R. Harte, X. Zhao, T. Carter, D. Grande, and J. A. Long. 2018. Effect of community health worker support on clinical outcomes of low-income patients across primary care facilities: A randomized clinical trial. *JAMA Internal Medicine* 178(12):1635-1643.

Kennedy, S., and L. Sheets. 2021. *Medicaid delivery system reforms to combat the opioid crisis.* Washington, DC: AcademyHealth.

Krishnamurti, T., A. L. Davis, B. Quinn, A. F. Castillo, K. L. Martin, and H. N. Simhan. 2021a. Mobile remote monitoring of intimate partner violence among pregnant patients during the COVID-19 shelter-in-place order: Quality improvement pilot study. *Journal of Medical Internet Research* 23(2):e22790.

Krishnamurti, T., A. L. Davis, S. Rodriguez, L. Hayani, M. Bernard, and H. N. Simhan. 2021b. Use of a smartphone app to explore potential underuse of prophylactic aspirin for preeclampsia. *JAMA Network Open* 4(10):e2130804.

Krishnamurti, T., M. Birru Talabi, L. S. Callegari, T. M. Kazmerski, and S. Borrero. 2022. A framework for FemTech: Guiding principles for developing digital reproductive health tools in the United States. *Journal of Medical Internet Research* 24(4):e36338.

Kwan, B. M., R. C. Brownson, R. E. Glasgow, E. H. Morrato, and D. A. Luke. 2022a. Designing for dissemination and sustainability to promote equitable impacts on health. *Annual Review of Public Health* 43:331-353.

Kwan, B. M., C. Sobczak, L. Beaty, M. K. Wynia, M. DeCamp, V. Owen, and A. A. Ginde. 2022b. Clinician perspectives on monoclonal antibody treatment for high-risk outpatients with COVID-19: Implications for implementation and equitable access. *Journal of General Internal Medicine* 37(13):3426-3434.

Lau, D., J. Soucie, J. Willits, S. H. Scholle, S. Kangovi, C. Garfield, and J. Feldstein. 2021. *Critical inputs for successful community health worker programs.* Washington, DC: National Committee for Quality Assurance.

Lee, K. C., A. U. Morgan, K. H. Chaiyachati, D. A. Asch, R. A. Xiong, D. Do, A. S. Kilaru, D. Lam, A. Parambath, A. B. Friedman, Z. F. Meisel, C. K. Snider, D. L. Chisholm, S. Kelly, J. E. Hemmons, D. Abdel-Rahman, J. Ebert, M. Ghosh, J. Reilly, C. J. O'Malley, L. Hahn, N. M. Mannion, A. M. Huffenberger, S. McGinley, M. Balachandran, N. Khan, J. A. Shea, N. Mitra, and M. K. Delgado. 2022. Pulse oximetry for monitoring patients with COVID-19 at home—a pragmatic, randomized trial. *New England Journal of Medicine* 386(19):1857-1859.

Maturo, A. M. 2012. Medicalization: Current concept and future directions in a bionic society. *Mens Sana Monographs* 10(1):122-133.

Mazzucca, S., E. M. Arredondo, D. M. Hoelscher, D. Haire-Joshu, R. G. Tabak, S. K. Kumanyika, and R. C. Brownson. 2021. Expanding implementation research to prevent chronic diseases in community settings. *Annual Review of Public Health* 42(1):135-158.

McCloskey, L. A., E. Lichter, C. Williams, M. Gerber, E. Wittenberg, and M. Ganz. 2006. Assessing intimate partner violence in health care settings leads to women's receipt of interventions and improved health. *Public Health Reports* 121(4):435-444.

McCormack, L., S. Sheridan, M. Lewis, V. Boudewyns, C. L. Melvin, C. Kistler, L. J. Lux, K. Cullen, and K. N. Lohr. 2013. Communication and dissemination strategies to facilitate the use of health-related evidence. *Evidence Report/Technology Assessment* (213):1-520.

Medicaid Outcomes Distributed Research Network. 2021. Use of medications for treatment of opioid use disorder among US Medicaid enrollees in 11 states, 2014-2018. *JAMA* 326(2):154-164.

Morgan, A. U., M. Balachandran, D. Do, D. Lam, A. Parambath, K. H. Chaiyachati, N. M. Bonalumi, S. C. Day, K. C. Lee, and D. A. Asch. 2020. Remote monitoring of patients with COVID-19: Design, implementation, and outcomes of the first 3,000 patients in COVID Watch. *NEJM Catalyst* July 21.

Morgan, A. U., D. T. Grande, T. Carter, J. A. Long, and S. Kangovi. 2016. Penn Center for Community Health Workers: Step-by-step approach to sustain an evidence-based community health worker intervention at an academic medical center. *American Journal of Public Health* 106(11):1958-1960.

Morehouse School of Medicine. 2022. *Office of Educational Outcomes and Assessment Guiding Principles.* https://www.msm.edu/oeoa/overview/Principles_Quality_Assessment.php (accessed September 28, 2022).

Morris, Z. S., S. Wooding, and J. Grant. 2011. The answer is 17 years, what is the question: Understanding time lags in translational research. *Journal of the Royal Society of Medicine* 104(12):510-520. doi: 10.1258/jrsm.2011.110180.

National Cancer Institute. 2004. *Making health communication programs work.* Washington, DC: National Cancer Institute.

NEJM (New England Journal of Medicine) Catalyst. 2017. *What Is Value-Based Healthcare?* https://catalyst.nejm.org/doi/full/10.1056/CAT.17.0558 (accessed September 14, 2022).

Nguyen, O. K., M. A. Vazquez, L. Charles, J. R. Berger, H. Quiñones, R. Fuquay, J. M. Sanders, K. A. Kapinos, E. A. Halm, and A. N. Makam. 2019. Association of scheduled vs emergency-only dialysis with health outcomes and costs in undocumented immigrants with end-stage renal disease. *JAMA Internal Medicine* 179(2):175-183.

Organizing Committee for Assessing Meaningful Community Engagement in Health & Health Care Programs & Policies. 2022. *Assessing meaningful community engagement: A conceptual model to advance health equity through transformed systems for health.* Washington, DC: National Academy of Medicine.

Phillips, R. L., N. F. Kanarek, and V. L. Boothe. 2021. Rebuilding a US federal data strategy after the end of the "community health status indicators." *American Journal of Public Health* 111(10):1865-1873.

Phillips, R. L., Jr., B. C. George, E. S. Holmboe, A. W. Bazemore, J. M. Westfall, and A. Bitton. 2022. Measuring graduate medical education outcomes to honor the social contract. *Academic Medicine* 97(5):643-648.

Podewils, L. J., T. L. Burket, C. Mettenbrink, A. Steiner, A. Seidel, K. Scott, L. Cervantes, and R. Hasnain-Wynia. 2020. Disproportionate incidence of COVID-19 infection, hospitalizations, and deaths among persons identifying as Hispanic or Latino—Denver, Colorado March-October 2020. *MMWR Morbidity and Mortality Weekly Report* 69(48):1812-1816.

Politi, M. C., C. N. Lee, S. E. Philpott-Streiff, R. E. Foraker, M. A. Olsen, C. Merrill, Y. Tao, and T. M. Myckatyn. 2020. A randomized controlled trial evaluating the BREASTchoice tool for personalized decision support about breast reconstruction after mastectomy. *Annals of Surgery* 271(2):230-237.

Ponder, M. L. 2022. What happens when the crisis seemingly never ends? Perspectives in health communication. *Ethnicity & Disease* 32(2):165-168.

Proctor, E., H. Silmere, R. Raghavan, P. Hovmand, G. Aarons, A. Bunger, R. Griffey, and M. Hensley. 2011. Outcomes for implementation research: Conceptual distinctions, measurement challenges, and research agenda. *Administration and Policy in Mental Health* 38(2):65-76.

Purtle, J., F. Lê-Scherban, X. Wang, P. T. Shattuck, E. K. Proctor, and R. C. Brownson. 2018. Audience segmentation to disseminate behavioral health evidence to legislators: An empirical clustering analysis. *Implementation Science* 13(1):1-13.

Purtle, J., F. Lê-Scherban, X. Wang, E. Brown, and M. Chilton. 2019a. State legislators' opinions about adverse childhood experiences as risk factors for adult behavioral health conditions. *Psychiatric Services* 70(10):894-900.

Purtle, J., F. Lê-Scherban, X. I. Wang, P. T. Shattuck, E. K. Proctor, and R. C. Brownson. 2019b. State legislators' support for behavioral health parity laws: The influence of mutable and fixed factors at multiple levels. *Milbank Quarterly* 97(4):1200-1232.

Purtle, J., J. S. Marzalik, R. W. Halfond, L. F. Bufka, B. A. Teachman, and G. A. Aarons. 2020. Toward the data-driven dissemination of findings from psychological science. *American Psychologist Journal* 75(8):1052-1066.

Purtle, J., K. L. Nelson, L. Gebrekristos, F. Lê-Scherban, and S. E. Gollust. 2022. Partisan differences in the effects of economic evidence and local data on legislator engagement with dissemination materials about behavioral health: A dissemination trial. *Implementation Science* 17(1):38.

Ramanathan, T., R. Hulkower, J. Holbrook, and M. Penn. 2017. Legal epidemiology: The science of law. *Journal of Law, Medicine & Ethics* 45(1_suppl):69-72.

Rossom, R. C., S. A. Hooker, P. J. O'Connor, A. L. Crain, and J. M. Sperl-Hillen. 2022. Cardiovascular risk for patients with and without schizophrenia, schizoaffective disorder, or bipolar disorder. *Journal of the American Heart Association* 11(6):e021444.

Schuster, J., C. Reynolds III, T. Carney, J. Kogan, C. Kang, P. Schake, and C. Nikolajski. 2019. *Using wellness coaches and extra support to improve the health and wellness of adults with serious mental illness.* Washington, DC: Patient-Centered Outcomes Research Institute.

Shearer, E. 2021. *More than eight-in-ten Americans get news from digital devices.* Washington, DC: Pew Research Center.

Shearer, E., and A. Mitchell. 2021. *News use across social media platforms in 2020.* Washington, DC: Pew Research Center.

Shelton, R. C., D. A. Chambers, and R. E. Glasgow. 2020. An extension of RE-AIM to enhance sustainability: Addressing dynamic context and promoting health equity over time. *Frontiers in Public Health* 8:134.

Shelton, R. C., L. E. Brotzman, D. Johnson, and D. Erwin. 2021. Trust and mistrust in shaping adaptation and de-implementation in the context of changing screening guidelines. *Ethnicity & Disease* 31(1):119-132.

Shukla, S., and S. Naganna. 2014. A review on K-means data clustering approach. *International Journal of Information and Computation Technology* 4(17):1847-1860.

Stewart, R. E., S. C. Marcus, T. R. Hadley, B. M. Hepburn, and D. S. Mandell. 2018. State adoption of incentives to promote evidence-based practices in behavioral health systems. *Psychiatric Services* 69(6):685-688.

Stock, C., S. Dias, T. Dietrich, A. Frasha, and I. Keygnaert. 2021. Editorial: How can we co-create solutions in health promotion with users and stakeholders? *Frontiers in Public Health* 9:773907.

Straube, B. M. 2009. Reform of the us healthcare system: Care of undocumented individuals with ESRD. *American Journal of Kidney Diseases* 53(6):921-924.

Swarbrick, M. 1997. A wellness model for clients. *Mental Health Special Interest Section Quarterly* 20(1):1-4.

Swarbrick, M. 2006. A wellness approach. *Psychiatric Rehabilitation Journal* 29(4):311-314.

Torous, J., S. Bucci, I. H. Bell, L. V. Kessing, M. Faurholt-Jepsen, P. Whelan, A. F. Carvalho, M. Keshavan, J. Linardon, and J. Firth. 2021. The growing field of digital psychiatry: Current evidence and the future of apps, social media, chatbots, and virtual reality. *World Psychiatry* 20(3):318-335.

Toye, C. R. A. 2016. Normalisation process theory and the implementation of resident assessment instrument–home care in Saskatchewan, Canada: A qualitative study. *Home Health Care Management & Practice* 28(3):161-169.

Vasan, A., J. W. Morgan, N. Mitra, C. Xu, J. A. Long, D. A. Asch, and S. Kangovi. 2020. Effects of a standardized community health worker intervention on hospitalization among disadvantaged patients with multiple chronic conditions: A pooled analysis of three clinical trials. *Health Services Research* 55(Suppl 2):894-901.

Westfall, J. M., R. Roper, A. Gaglioti, and D. E. Nease, Jr. 2019. Practice-based research networks: Strategic opportunities to advance implementation research for health equity. *Ethnicity & Disease* 29(Suppl 1):113-118.

WHO (World Health Organization). 2018a. *Guidelines for the management of physical health conditions in adults with severe mental disorders.* Geneva, Switzerland: World Health Organization.

WHO. 2018b. *WHO guideline on health policy and system support to optimize community health worker programmes.* Geneva: World Health Organization.

Wong, I. H., and T. T. Wong. 2021. Exploring the relationship between intellectual humility and academic performance among post-secondary students: The mediating roles of learning motivation and receptivity to feedback. *Learning and Individual Differences* 88:102012.

Xu, T. T., F. Zhou, C. Y. Deng, G. Q. Huang, J. K. Li, and X. D. Wang. 2015. Low-dose aspirin for preventing preeclampsia and its complications: A meta-analysis. *Journal of Clinical Hypertension (Greenwich)* 17(7):567-573.

Zechner, M., M. Swarbrick, M. Fullen, N. Barrett, S. Santos-Tuano, and C. Pratt. 2021. Wellness for OA 1 multi-dimensional wellness for people aging with mental health conditions: A proposed framework. *Psychiatric Rehabilitation Journal* 45(2):160-169.

Zivin, K., L. Allen, A. J. Barnes, S. Junker, J. Y. Kim, L. Tang, S. Kennedy, K. A. Ahrens, M. Burns, S. Clark, E. Cole, D. Crane, D. Idala, P. Lanier, S. Mohamoud, M. Jarlenski, M. J. McDuffie, J. Talbert, A. J. Gordon, and J. M. Donohue. 2022. Design, implementation, and evolution of the Medicaid Outcomes Distributed Research Network (MODRN). *Medical Care* 60(9):680-690.

Appendix A

Statement of Task

A planning committee of the National Academies of Sciences, Engineering, and Medicine (the National Academies) will plan and host a series of four public workshops to explore potential ways for the Agency for Healthcare Research and Quality (AHRQ) to accelerate the use of patient-centered outcomes research (PCOR) findings in clinical practice to improve health and health care. The workshops will feature invited presentations and discussions examining topics in four main categories:

1. Ways to revise and improve the AHRQ's proposed strategic plan, priorities, and strategies to make them clearer and more likely to lead to funding high impact and complementary projects while being consistent with the congressional mandate for investing funds from the PCOR Trust Fund (PCORTF), e.g.,
   - Opportunities to train and educate PCOR investigators, while also addressing AHRQ's PCORTF strategic priorities
   - Development of digital tools to increase implementation of PCOR findings into practice
   - Sustainable strategies for expanding implementation of PCOR findings
   - The potential for development of an overall coordinated interdisciplinary approach to decisions about AHRQ's PCORTF investments
2. Ways to measure progress and the impact of AHRQ's PCORTF

investments as a whole on meeting its goals (in the short term, proximate, and long term). For example:
- Currently available metrics,
- Currently available data sources,
- Potential for novel metrics, analytics, and data sources, and
- Ways to harmonize data elements across projects that could be included in evaluating the short- and long-term impact of AHRQ's PCORTF investments.

3. Ways to better align priorities and strategies and to create complementary collaborations between the agencies charged with using the PCORTF to improve patient-centered outcomes research and practice (AHRQ, PCORI and ASPE), so as to increase the impact of AHRQ's PCORTF investments and their potential to sustainably reduce disparities.
4. Ways AHRQ can apply communication science to improve dissemination of evidence, gaps in evidence, and policy gaps to inform health policies and decision-makers at the local, state, and federal levels.

The planning committee, with support from National Academies staff, will organize the workshop, select and invite speakers and discussants, and moderate the discussions. A proceedings of the presentations and discussions at the workshops will be prepared by a designated rapporteur in accordance with institutional guidelines.

Appendix B

Workshop Agendas

VIRTUAL WORKSHOP 1, THURSDAY JUNE 9, 2022

8:00–8:15am **Welcome and Workshop Overview**
Lauren Hughes, Planning Committee Chair, University of Colorado

Sponsor Remarks from AHRQ
Karin Rhodes, Chief Implementation Officer

8:15–8:45am **IMPaCT: A Person-Centered Community Health Worker Model**
Moderator: Lauren Hughes, Planning Committee Chair, University of Colorado
Speakers:
- Shreya Kangovi, University of Pennsylvania
- Brea Burke, Healing Hands Health Center

8:45–8:55am **Break**

8:55–9:50am   Session 1: Developing a Coordinated Interdisciplinary Approach to Decision Making Around Where to Focus AHRQ's PCORTF Investments
Moderator: Catherine Kothari, Western Michigan University Homer Stryker MD School of Medicine
Speakers:
- Reshma Gupta, University of California, Davis
- Donald Nease, University of Colorado

Panel Discussion

9:50–10:05am   Break

10:05–11:00am   Session 2: Training PCOR Investigators
Moderator: Meghan Lane-Fall, University of Pennsylvania
Speakers:
- Nivedita Mohanty, Alliance Chicago
- Cynthia Gonzalez, Charles Drew University, RAND Corporation

Panel Discussion / Q & A

11:00–11:15am   Break

11:15am–12:20pm   Session 3: Sustainable Strategies and Digital Tools to Expand Implementation of PCOR Findings
Moderator: Cara Nikolajski, University of Pittsburgh Medical Center
Speakers:
- James Schuster, University of Pittsburgh Medical Center
- Tamar Krishnamurti, University of Pittsburgh
- Andrea Graham, Northwestern University

Panel Discussion / Q & A

12:20–12:30pm   Recap and Adjourn
Lauren Hughes, Planning Committee Chair, University of Colorado

APPENDIX B

VIRTUAL WORKSHOP 2 FRIDAY JUNE 17, 2022

8:00–8:15am **Welcome and Workshop Overview**
Lauren Hughes, Planning Committee Chair, University of Colorado

Sponsor Remarks from AHRQ
Karin Rhodes, Chief Implementation Officer, AHRQ

8:15–8:45am **Centering Equity in PCOR Through Meaningful Community Engagement**
Moderator: Jen Brown, Northwestern University
Speaker: Sergio Aguilar-Gaxiola, University of California Davis Health

8:55–9:05am Break

9:05-10:35am **Session 1: Possibilities for AHRQ-ASPE-PCORI Collaborations to Improve Health Equity**
Moderator: Brian Rivers, Morehouse School of Medicine
Speakers:
- Gary Puckrein, National Minority Quality Forum
- Anne Gaglioti, MetroHealth System, Morehouse School of Medicine
- Rachel Shelton, Columbia University, Mailman School of Public Health
- George Rust, Florida State University

Panel Discussion

10:35–10:50am Break

10:50am–12:20pm **Session 2: Opportunities for AHRQ-ASPE-PCORI Collaborations to Improve Sustainability of Their Efforts**
Moderator: Megan Daugherty Douglas, Morehouse School of Medicine
Speakers:
- Abby Collier, National Center for Fatality Review and Prevention
- Lynn Blewett, Ph.D., University of Minnesota
- Robert L. Phillips Jr., American Board of Family Medicine

	Panel Discussion
12:20pm	**Recap and Adjourn** Lauren Hughes, Planning Committee Chair, University of Colorado

VIRTUAL WORKSHOP 3 FRIDAY JULY 1, 2022

8:00–8:15am	**Welcome and Workshop Overview** Lauren Hughes, Planning Committee Chair, University of Colorado
	Sponsor Remarks from AHRQ Karin Rhodes, Chief Implementation Officer
8:15–9:45am	**Measuring the Impact of Dissemination and Implementation** Projects Part 1 *Moderator:* Brian Rivers, Morehouse School of Medicine *Speakers:* • Karen Glanz, University of Pennsylvania • Silas Buchanan, Institute for E- Health Equity • Bethany M. Kwan, University of Colorado
9:45–10:00am	Break
10:00–11:30am	**Measuring the Impact of Dissemination and Implementation** Projects Part 2 *Moderator:* Sarah Scholle, National Committee for Quality Assurance *Speakers:* • Alisa J. Stephens-Shields, University of Pennsylvania • Mary Politi, Washington University in St. Louis • Krisda Chaiyachati, Verify Health
	Panel Discussion / Q & A
11:30am	**Closing Remarks**

APPENDIX B

VIRTUAL WORKSHOP 4 WEDNESDAY JULY 6, 2022

8:00–8:15am **Welcome and Workshop Overview**
Lauren Hughes, Planning Committee Chair, University of Colorado
Sponsor Remarks from AHRQ
Karin Rhodes, Chief Implementation Officer

8:15–9:45am **Session 1 Effective Communication Tools**
Moderator: Cara Nikolajski, University of Pittsburgh Medical Center
Speakers:
- Manisha Sharma, CentiVox Media Group & Community Health Group
- Monica Ponder, Howard University
- Dawn Hunter, Network for Public Health

Panel Discussion

9:45–10:00am Break

10:00–11:35am **Session 2 Informing Evidence-Based Policy Making**
Moderator: Lauren Hughes, University of Colorado
Speakers:
- Renuka Tipirneni, University of Michigan (Pre-recorded presentation)
- Lilia Cervantes, University of Colorado
- Jonathan Purtle, NYU

Panel Discussion / Q & A

11:35am Recap and Adjourn

APPENDIX C

Biographical Sketches of the Speakers

Sergio Aguilar-Gaxiola, M.D., Ph.D., is an internationally renowned expert on mental health in ethnic populations. As on-site principal investigator of the Mexican American Prevalence and Services Survey—the largest mental health study conducted in the United States on Mexican Americans—he identified the most prevalent mental health disorders in the Mexican-origin population in California's central valley; showed that the rate of disorders increases the longer the individual resides in the United States; and demonstrated that children of immigrants have even greater rates of mental disorders. From this study, he developed a model of service delivery that increased access to mental health services among the Central Valley's low-income, underserved, rural populations. Dr. Aguilar-Gaxiola conducts cross-national epidemiologic studies on the patterns and correlates of psychiatric disorders in general population samples. He is the coordinator for Latin America and the Caribbean of the World Health Organization's Mental Health Survey, and coordinates the work of the National Mental Health Institute surveys in Mexico, Columbia, Brazil, Peru, Costa Rica, and Portugal. He also develops culturally and linguistically sensitive diagnostic mental health measures, and translates mental health research into practical information for consumers and their families, health professionals, service administrators, and policy makers.

Silas Buchanan is an experienced underserved community outreach and engagement strategist. He is the founding CEO of the Institute for eHealth Equity where he leads partnerships with health care payer, provider, pharma, life sciences, medical device, government, and academic stakeholders. Mr.

Buchanan has expertise in crafting web-based ecosystems that solve for known, underserved community outreach and engagement failure points. He recently launched OurHealthMinistry.com in partnership with Morehouse School of Medicine, and co-developed AMECHealth.org as the official health information-sharing channel for the AME Church, the largest mainline, historically Black denomination in the world (2,000 congregations/2 million members). Mr. Buchanan currently works closely with the Milken Institute, FasterCures Workgroup on DEI in Clinical Trials, the American Telemedicine Workgroup on Eliminating Health Disparities, and the Digital Medicine Society Data Steering Committee. He has contributed thought leadership to HIMSS, Accenture, National Academy of Medicine, the Clinical Trials Transformation Initiative, and the Harvard Business School, Kraft Precision Medicine Accelerator. Mr. Buchanan has testified before the HHS, HIT Policy Committee. He was selected as member of the White House Summit to Achieve eHealth Equity and selected as co-chair of the Awareness Committee for Region V of the HHS National Partnership for Action to End Health Disparities. He is an Inaugural member of the National eHealth Collaborative Consumer Committee and is a member of the Ohio Patient-Centered Primary Care Collaborative.

Brea Burke is a trained community health worker through Penn's Center for CHW. She is a Virginia Certified CHW and has also received training through the Institute for Public Health Innovation. She has spoken about the work of CHWs for numerous virtual workshops and was a guest on the the National Center for Quality Assurance podcast discussing the importance of CHWs in both rural and larger communities. She was recently interviewed by *The Atlantic* about the importance of CHWs and their pivotal role in seeing their communities through the pandemic. Ms. Burke is the founder and leader of the CHWUnited group of Southwest Virginia and Northeast Tennessee. She is a member of CHAMPP (Community Health Workers Advocating for Movement in Policy and Practice), the Bristol VA/Bristol TN Community Homeless Coalition, and the Community Based Workforce Alliance policy workgroup.

Lilia Cervantes, M.D., is the director of immigrant health and an associate professor in the Department of Medicine at the University of Colorado (CU) Anschutz Medical Campus. Dr. Cervantes received her undergraduate degree at CU Boulder and completed her medical degree and internal medicine residency at the University of Colorado School of Medicine. Dr. Cervantes is recognized for spearheading an innovative change to a Medicaid payment rule in Colorado to give undocumented patients with kidney failure access to life-saving maintenance dialysis. The collaborative effort came after the passing of her patient and friend, Hilda, a young mother of two boys who was ineligible for routine dialysis due to her undocumented status. Her loss was life-changing for Dr. Cervantes, and she coped with the loss through commitment and action. Through strategic documentation and dissection of the enormous human and economic costs of the status quo, and through grit and persistence, Dr. Cervantes conducted research, developed a coalition of allies, and a policy remedy to save others like Hilda. The efforts have garnered national attention and partnerships, leading, in turn, to efforts to enable routine dialysis for underserved patients in several other states. Following this defining experience, Dr. Cervantes's work has focused on eliminating structural racism in kidney health disparities. Dr. Cervantes conducted mixed-methods studies to understand the social challenges and perspectives of Latinx with kidney failure and in partnership with a community advisory panel, translated her findings to create community-based interventions. Dr. Cervantes has received over 15 awards for her service to her community and is a member of nine civic and community activity boards.

Krisda Chaiyachati, M.D., M.P.H., M.S.H.P., is the physician lead for value-based care and innovation for Verily Health Platforms at Verily, an Alphabet company and formerly Google Life Sciences, a division of Google X. He is a physician executive with extensive background in health care innovation, health services research, epidemiology, and health policy with a lens toward the role of health care technology in transforming care delivery to make it more efficient, equitable, and accessible. He has led the development and evaluation of telemedicine, artificial intelligence, or automation in health care. He has published over 60 peer-reviewed articles and is a coauthor of an upcoming book, *Seems Like a Good Idea: Evidence-Based Innovation in Medical Care Delivery and Financing*. Prior to Verily, Dr. Chaiyachati held leadership roles at the University of Pennsylvania Health System as the medical director for Penn Medicine OnDemand Virtual Care, the medical director for PennOpen Pass, and the director for the Leonard Davis Institute-Penn Medicine Research Laboratory. Dr. Chaiyachati completed his internal medicine training in Yale's Primary Care Residency Program where he served as a chief resident. In addition to his medical degree from the University of Michigan, Dr. Chaiyachati holds a master's degree in public health from the Harvard School of Public Health, and a master's degree in health policy research from the University of Pennsylvania as a Robert Wood Johnson Clinical Scholar.

Abby Collier, M.S., is the director at the National Center for Fatality Review and Prevention (National Center), a program of MPHI. In this role, Ms. Collier leads the National Center in providing technical assistance and support to local and state child death review and fetal infant mortality review programs throughout the United States. Additionally, Ms. Collier oversees the National

Fatality Review-Case Reporting System (NFR-CRS), which is used by child death review and fetal infant mortality review teams in 47 states. NFR-CRS captures information about how and why children die to help prevent future deaths. Ms. Collier provides training and technical assistance on a wide variety of topics including best practices in fatality review, reducing secondary trauma, improving data quality, improving equity in fatality review, and building partnerships. Ms. Collier has a master's degree in counseling and is pursuing a doctorate in public health.

Anne Gaglioti, M.D., M.S., FAAFP, is a family physician and serves as an associate professor at the Population Health Research Institute at The Metro-Health System and Case Western Reserve University and the Center for Community Health Integration at Case Western Reserve University in Cleveland, Ohio. She is a senior strategic adviser and associate professor at the National Center for Primary Care at Morehouse School of Medicine in Atlanta, Georgia. She is originally from Cleveland, Ohio, and completed her medical school and residency training in family medicine at Case Western Reserve University and completed fellowship training in primary care health policy and research at Georgetown University and the Robert Graham Center for Policy Studies in Washington, DC. She received her master of science degree in clinical research at Morehouse School of Medicine. Her academic career as a teacher and researcher has been focused on advancing equity, patient and stakeholder engaged research infrastructure, and measurement of the impact the primary care system has on health and health equity. As co-director of the Southeast Regional Clinicians Network, a practice-based research network made up of Federally Qualified Health Centers across eight southeastern states, she conducts practice-based research in the primary care safety net grounded in a robust patient and stakeholder engagement infrastructure. She is also a health services researcher and her work with health care claims and other large data sets focuses on the intersection of primary care, place, and health equity among populations disproportionately impacted by health inequities.

Karen Glanz, Ph.D., M.P.H., is George A. Weiss University Professor, and professor in the Perelman School of Medicine and the School of Nursing at the University of Pennsylvania (UPenn). She is associate director for community-engaged research and program co-leader for the cancer control program at the Abramson Cancer Center at UPenn. Her research in community and health care settings focuses on obesity, nutrition, and the built environment; reducing health disparities; dissemination and implementation science; and health communication technologies. She has published over 540 articles and chapters and is lead editor on five editions of the widely used text, Health Behavior: Theory, Research and Practice (Jossey-Bass: 1990, 1996, 2002, 2008, 2015).

Dr. Glanz was elected to membership in the National Academy of Medicine of the National Academy of Sciences in 2013.

Cynthia Gonzalez, Ph.D., M.P.H., is a first-generation Mexican American lifetime resident of Watts that brings a strong background in community-based participatory research, cultural anthropology, and social ethnography to the understanding of community wellness. Influenced by her upbringing, Dr. Gonzalez is interested in participatory research as a tool for equity, social justice, and critical multidisciplinary scholarship. She has developed partnerships between community, government, and academia and has served as a community adviser to numerous place-based and racial justice focused projects. As the former senior project manager of the Watts Rising Collaborative, she led a multi-million-dollar infrastructure grant for the Housing Authority of the City of Los Angeles. Most recently, Dr. Gonzalez serves as the director of the Pardee RAND Graduate School's Community-Partnered Policy and Action Stream Ph.D. program in policy analysis where students prepare to be future scholars that are mindful of how social dynamics impact research, using an equity and racial justice lens. In addition, Dr. Gonzalez is an assistant professor in the M.P.H. Program in Urban Health at Charles R. Drew University of Medicine and Science and currently advises on COVID-19 related projects to ensure local community representation and inclusion. She leads a COVID-19 education project for mental health clinicians serving communities like where she grew up. Dr. Gonzalez graduated UCLA with a B.A. in Chicana/o studies and public health, completed an M.P.H. in biostatistics and epidemiology from USC and a Ph.D. in social and cultural anthropology from the California Institute of Integral Studies.

Andrea Graham, Ph.D., is assistant professor in the Center for Behavioral Intervention Technologies at Northwestern University's Feinberg School of Medicine, with an affiliation in the Center for Human-Computer Interaction + Design. Trained as a clinical psychologist and implementation scientist, her program of research focuses on the design, optimization, and implementation of evidence-based digital mental and behavioral health interventions. She is a leader in applying human-centered design methods to design digital tools that meet stakeholders' needs and implementation plans that support the integration of digital interventions into practice. She also has expertise in designing and overseeing coaching protocols and clinical workflows for digital interventions.

Reshma Gupta, M.D., M.S.H.P.M., is a practicing internist, the chief of population health and accountable care at University of California Davis Health in Sacramento, CA, and part of the Population Health Leadership Team for strategy across all UC Health campuses. She is a creative physician-leader with executive management experience in clinical and operational strategy, quality improvement, digital health, and care model design. Dr. Gupta has been featured as a Top Executive Population Health Leader in Becker's Hospital Review. She has led hundreds of clinician and care team members in population health and affordability improvement initiatives, linking initiatives to trainee education, and managing health system value analytics through a learning health system model. Dr. Gupta's work has focused on health system innovation, policy, and implementation to better define and improve the culture of delivering more affordable care to patients. She has worked as a senior adviser with the Center for Medicare and Medicaid Innovations' Comprehensive Primary Care program to test new models of value promoting payment reform. Her research created the first High-Value Care Culture Survey, evaluated drivers of value-based decision-making in medical centers across California, and evaluated interventions to reduce expenditures for high-cost conditions. She serves as a senior adviser of Costs of Care where she leads a learning community of over 500 health system managers and educators across six countries. Dr. Gupta has consulted and speaks nationally on population health and health care affordability. She has published in journals such as the *JAMA, Health Affairs, NEJM Catalyst, Journal of General and Internal Medicine, Academic Medicine*, and media outlets including NPR, CNN, and ABC NewsRadio. Dr. Gupta received a bachelor's degree from UC Berkeley and doctor of medicine degree from UC San Francisco. She completed her residency and chief residency in internal medicine at the University of Washington Seattle and the Robert Wood Johnson Clinical Scholar Fellowship and Masters in Health Policy and Management at UCLA. She is a distinguished leader of the California Health Care Foundation and Presidential Leadership Scholars programs.

Dawn Hunter, J.D., M.P.H., is director of the Southeastern Region of the Network for Public Health Law. She is an experienced state health department policy maker and legislative director whose work focuses on research, analysis, implementation, and capacity building related to the use of law and policy to improve health outcomes and advance racial equity. She previously served as deputy state health official in New Mexico, where she led legislative planning and policy development, strategic planning, performance management, and public health accreditation. Currently, Ms. Hunter leads an ongoing assessment of declarations of racism as a public health crisis and related efforts to address health inequities. She also focuses on strategies to improve health outcomes through civic engagement and conducts training on equity in public health messaging. Ms. Hunter started her career in child protective services in Hillsborough County, Florida. She later transitioned into research and development as a microbiologist at the USF Center for Biological Defense before embarking on her current path. Ms. Hunter is certified in public health by the National Board of Public Health Examiners. She received her A.B. in English literature from Princeton University, her B.S. in microbiology and her M.P.H. in global communicable disease from the University of South Florida, and her J.D. from Stetson University College of Law.

Shreya Kangovi, M.D., M.S., founding executive director of the Penn Center for Community Health Workers, and an associate professor at the University of Pennsylvania Perelman School of Medicine, is a leading expert on improving population health through evidence-based community health worker (CHW) programs. Dr. Kangovi founded the Penn Center for CHWs, a national center of excellence dedicated to advancing health in low-income populations through effective CHW programs. She has authored numerous scientific publications and received over $25 million in funding, including federal grants from the National Institutes of Health and the Patient-Centered Outcomes Research Institute. She is the recipient of the 2019 Robert Wood Johnson Foundation Health Equity Award, an elected member of the American College of Physicians, and a member of the National Academies of Sciences, Engineering, and Medicine's Roundtable on the Promotion of Health Equity.

Tamar Krishnamurti, Ph.D., is an assistant professor of medicine and clinical and translational science at the University of Pittsburgh. Dr. Krishnamurti draws on (and develops) methods in the social and decision sciences, working with cross-disciplinary experts and community, to examine issues at the intersection of health, risk, technology, and the environment. Dr. Krishnamurti was the recipient of S&R Foundation's 2020 Kuno Award for Applied Science to develop mobile health strategies to identify and intervene on maternal health risks. She is a co-founder of the FemTech Collaborative, housed within the University of Pittsburgh's Center for Innovative Research on Gender Health Equity.

Nivedita Mohanty, M.D., is the chief research officer at AllianceChicago. Dr. Mohanty is a board-certified pediatrician with 15 years of experience in community health, clinical research, academic medicine, and international volunteerism. AllianceChicago is a national network of over 50 Federally Qualified Health Centers (FQHCs) across 19 states and a Practice-Based Research Network. Dr. Mohanty joined AllianceChicago in 2015 after spending a year in Washington, DC, as an American Association for the Advancement of Science Fellow in the Smart and Connected Health program, a program jointly supported by the National Science Foundation and National Institutes of Health (NIH). As a fellow within a federal agency, she gained firsthand exposure to the synergies health services research, clinical practice, and policy and the role of Health Information Technology (HIT) in advancing national health priorities. Dr. Mohanty works closely with FQHCs to leverage AllianceChicago's HIT infrastructure and strategic partnerships to support high-quality care in community health and the generation of new and relevant evidence through community-driven research. She has led the implementation and community engagement for multiple clinical trials funded by the Patient-Centered Outcomes Research Institute, the Agency for Healthcare Research and Quality, and NIH. Dr. Mohanty is a clinical associate professor at the Northwestern University Feinberg School of Medicine and continues to provide patient care at Erie Family Health Center and Ann and Robert Lurie Children's Hospital in Chicago. Dr. Mohanty has served families in 10 countries on numerous international medical initiatives with organization such as Operation Smile, Rotaplast International, and the International Children's Heart Foundation.

Donald E. Nease, Jr., M.D., is a professor of family medicine at the University of Colorado Anschutz Medical Campus, where he serves as the Green-Edelman Chair for Practice-Based Research, director of community engagement for the Colorado Clinical and Translational Sciences Institute, vice chair for community in the Department of Family Medicine and director of the SNOCAP Practice-Based Research Network Collaborative. He completed his undergraduate degree and medical school at the University of Kansas, residency at the Medical University of South Carolina in Charleston, and a Faculty Development Fellowship at the University of North Carolina at Chapel Hill. Dr. Nease's passion is to improve health in partnership with communities, patients, and clinicians and their practices. He works this territory from the level of individual interactions to community- and population-based interventions.

Robert L. Phillips, Jr., M.D., M.S.P.H., is a graduate of the Missouri University of Science and Technology and the University of Florida College of Medicine where he graduated with honors for special distinction. He trained in family medicine at the University of Missouri, followed by a fellowship in health services research and public health. Dr. Phillips was the director of the Robert Graham Center in Washington, DC, from 2004–2012. In 2012, he moved to the American Board of Family Medicine as vice president for research and policy and in 2018, Dr. Phillips was named the founding executive director of the Center for Professionalism and Value in Health Care. Dr. Phillips currently practices part time in a community-based residency program and is a professor of family medicine at Georgetown University and Virginia Commonwealth University. He also has faculty appointments at George Washington University and Harvard Medical School. He previously served on the American Medical Association's Council on Medical Education, as president of the National Residency Matching Program, vice chair of the U.S. Council on Graduate Medical Education, and co-chair of population health on the National Committee for Vital and Health Statistics. He served as a Fulbright Specialist to the Netherlands in 2012 and New Zealand in 2016. A nationally recognized leader on primary care policy and health care reform, Dr. Phillips was elected to the National Academy of Medicine in 2010 and currently chairs the NAM Membership Committee.

Mary C. Politi, Ph.D., is a professor in the Department of Surgery, Division of Public Health Sciences at Washington University in St. Louis School of Medicine. Dr. Politi's primary research interests include health communication and shared decision-making. Her work helps patients and the public understand health information, explore what is important to them when making health decisions, and collaborate to make evidence-informed decisions that meet their needs. She also trains health care professionals, public health advocates, and members of the public interested in shared decision-making and patient engagement. Dr. Politi's research includes a focus on reducing health disparities by engaging communities with unmet health needs and including them in both research and dissemination efforts. She works extensively with stakeholders to ensure her research is relevant to end users in clinical and community settings.

Monica Ponder, Ph.D., M.S.P.H., is an assistant professor of health communication and culture in the Cathy Hughes School of Communication at Howard University. Dr. Ponder's research interests are focused on organization-level health and crisis communication practice. She is the co-lead of Project REFOCUS (Racial Ethnic Framing of Community-Informed and Unifying Surveillance), an initiative that addresses social stigma related to COVID-19 and racism. Dr. Ponder is also the creator of The Henrietta Hypothesis, an interdisciplinary model for crisis communication. It is a 16-construct model aptly named "*The Henrietta Hypothesis*" in honor of Henrietta Lacks' iconic health care case. This scholarship offers crisis communication recommendations for public health organizations seeking to understand, reach, and engage historically marginalized and underrepresented groups during public health emergencies. As a scholar activist, Dr. Ponder has led many successful public health initiatives including advocating for the establishment of lactation rooms (pods) at Hartsfield-Jackson Atlanta International Airport—the world's busiest airport, as well as leading plans for lactation support services for the 2017 National Women's March (Washington, DC). As a lifelong learner and practitioner, Dr. Ponder leverages, in her teaching, her 10+ year career in health communication at the Centers for Disease Control and Prevention. Dr. Ponder views the classroom as a safe space and hopes that, through this process, students become aware of their own power as scholar activists, empowered learners, and as emerging public health change-makers. Dr. Ponder holds B.S. and M.S. degrees in chemistry from Clark Atlanta University, an M.S.P.H. in epidemiology from Emory University and a Ph.D. in communication from Georgia State University.

Gary A. Puckrein, Ph.D., is the founding president and chief executive officer of the National Minority Quality Forum (NMQF), a nonprofit health care research, education, and advocacy organization headquartered in Washington, DC. The mission of NMQF is to reduce patient risk by assuring optimal care for all. NMQF conducts evidence-based, data-driven initiatives to eliminate premature death and preventable illness. NMQF's vision is an American health services research, delivery, and financing system whose operating principle is to reduce patient risk for amenable morbidity and mortality while improving quality of life. Dr. Puckrein received his doctorate from Brown University.

Jonathan Purtle, Dr.P.H., M.P.H., is associate professor of public health policy and management and director of policy research at New York University's Global Center for Implementation Science. Dr. Purtle is an implementation scientist whose research focuses on mental health policy. His work examines questions such as how research evidence can be most effectively communicated to policy makers and is used in policy-making processes, how social and political contexts affect policy making and policy implementation, and how the implementation of policies "on the books" can be improved in practice. He is also interested in population-based approaches to mental health and how mental health can be integrated into mainstream public health practice. Dr. Purtle's work has been consistently funded by the National Institute of Mental Health (NIMH) and Robert Wood Johnson Foundation (RWJF). He is currently leading NIMH-funded projects focused on the implementation of policies that earmark taxes for mental health services and understanding the dynamics of research evidence in mental health policy making and a RWJF-funded project that experimentally tests different ways of communicating evidence about child maltreatment to the public and policy makers. His research is regularly published in journals such as *Implementation Science, Psychiatric Services, The Milbank Quarterly,* and *Annual Review of Public Health.* He has been the chair of the policy section of the AcademyHealth/NIH Dissemination and Implementation in Health Conference since 2017 and was awarded the 2018 Champion of Evidence-Based Interventions Award from the Association for Behavioral and Cognitive Therapies for his work on evidence use in mental health policy making.

George Rust, M.D., M.P.H., FAAFP, FACPM, is a professor at the Florida State University College of Medicine in Tallahassee, FL, where he also directs the Center for Medicine and Public Health. He also serves as medical executive director for the Leon County Health Department and five surrounding rural counties. He is board-certified in both family practice and in preventive medicine. He completed a family medicine residency at Cook County Hospital in Chicago, and then began his career serving 6 years as medical director for the West Orange Farmworkers Health Association in Central Florida, where he developed innovative community programs such as the diabetic promotora project. He then taught for 24 years on faculty at the Morehouse School of Medicine, where he was founding director of the Morehouse Faculty Development Program as well as the National Center for Primary Care. He also served as lead author for the Georgia Health Disparities Report plus Hispanic and Asian health disparity supplements. He was a key leader in an academic-private partnership for population health management that was estimated to have saved Georgia Medicaid over $100 million. In 2015, he was senior scientific adviser to the U.S. Agency for Healthcare Research and Quality. As a population health outcomes and health equity researcher, Dr. Rust has authored over 120 peer-reviewed publications, and has received numerous local, state, and national awards for teaching and service. His career as a family physician and scholar has consistently focused on primary health care and community health for those in greatest need, and on charting a path to health equity.

James Schuster, M.D., M.B.A., is the chief medical officer for the University of Pittsburgh Medical Center (UPMC) Insurance Services Division where he has served in leadership roles for nearly two decades. In addition, Dr. Schuster oversees the UPMC Center for High-Value Healthcare which has an extensive record of multiple research awards and publications and he is a member of the Board of Governors of the Patient-Centered Outcomes Research Institute. Dr. Schuster received his undergraduate degree at Washington University in St. Louis. He completed his medical education at the University of Louisville and his residency in psychiatry and an M.B.A. at the University of Pittsburgh. He is currently a clinical professor in the University of Pittsburgh Department of Psychiatry and has an extensive record of publications. He also has board certifications in general, addictions, and geriatric psychiatry.

Manisha Sharma, M.D., FAAFP, is a board-certified family medicine physician who works at the intersection of health justice and equity, patient care, health policy, system design, and clinical innovation. Dr. Sharma leads and provides strategic advisory support on multiple local, state, and national initiatives geared to dismantle structural racism in medicine and end health inequities. She appears often on several major television networks, including NBC, MSNBC, CNN, CBS, and Fox News addressing topics such as health and racial equity, health in all policy, social justice, wellness, and health. She has organized and led numerous grassroots physician campaigns through the organization Doctors for America where she served as the national director of leadership cultivation. She is the senior medical director of Community Health Group and a recent graduate of the California Health Care Foundation Leadership and Innovation Fellowship. She is a co-founder of Civic Health Alliance (a nonpartisan coalition of health professionals and students, committed to helping peers and patients register to vote and vote safely), and CentiVox Media Group, a social impact firm that transforms public health communications by elevating health care providers, scientists, and health and equity experts as trusted messengers.

Rachel C. Shelton, Sc.D., M.P.H., is a social and behavioral scientist with training in cancer and social epidemiology, and expertise in implementation science, sustainability, health equity, and community-based participatory research. She is associate professor of sociomedical sciences at Columbia University's Mailman School of Public Health, where she is co-director of the Community Engagement Core Resource at the Irving Institute for Clinical and Translational Research (CTSA), and is director of a university-wide Implementation Science Initiative. Dr. Shelton has taught implementation science courses and trainings nationally and globally for nearly 10 years, including TIDIRC, TIDIRH, and the Institute for Implementation Science Scholars. Dr. Shelton has 15 years of experience conducting mixed-methods research focused on advancing the implementation and sustainability of evidence-based interventions in community and clinical settings to address health inequities, particularly in the context of cancer prevention/control; her research program is funded by NIA, NCI, NIMHD and American Cancer Society.

Alisa J. Stephens-Shields, Ph.D., is an associate professor of biostatistics at the University of Pennsylvania Perelman School of Medicine. Her research focuses on extensions and innovative applications of causal inference to enhance the design and analysis of clinical trials. She also works in the development of patient-reported outcomes to inform population-appropriate trial endpoints. Dr. Stephens-Shields collaborates in several areas, including pediatrics, pharmacoepidemiology, behavioral economics, and implementation science. She is currently the lead statistical investigator for the Handoffs and Transitions in Critical Care–Understanding Scalability study, a stepped wedge randomized trial aiming to improve patient outcomes through designing and implementing standardized, tailored protocols for transitioning patients from operating rooms to intensive care units, and the recently American Heart Association-awarded Behavioral Economics to Transform Trial Enrollment Representativeness Center, which will evaluate methods to increase diverse participation in clinical trials. Dr. Stephens-Shields was a recipient of the inaugural Committee of Presidents of Statistical Societies Leadership Academy award and currently serves as an associate editor of *Biostatistics* and a statistical consultant for the *Annals of Internal Medicine*. She holds Ph.D. and A.M. degrees in biostatistics from Harvard University and a B.S. in mathematics with minor in Spanish from the University of Maryland, College Park.

Renuka Tipirneni, M.D., M.Sc., is an assistant professor in the Department of Internal Medicine, Divisions of General Medicine and Hospital Medicine, and serves as faculty adviser to the Policy Engagement Team at the Institute for Healthcare Policy and Innovation (IHPI) at the University of Michigan. Her research focuses on investigating the impact of health reform policies and programs on low socioeconomic status, minority, aging, and other vulnerable populations, and on delivery of care in the health care safety net. Her current work includes examinations of Medicaid policy, Medicare and other health reform policy for older adults, and integration of social determinants of health into clinical practice. She has evaluated the Affordable Care Act, Michigan's Medicaid expansion, and other state and federal policies, and is a recipient of a K08 career development award from the National Institute on Aging for her work examining the impact of coverage expansions on near retirement adults. Dr. Tipirneni is passionate about the translation of research into implementation of health policies and health care delivery, including sharing lessons learned across communities and states.

Appendix D

AHRQ's PCORTF Investment Strategic Framework

Strategic Framework to Guide AHRQ's PCORTF Investments

Mission:	Overarching Vision:	High-level Goal:
Synthesize and support the dissemination of evidence into practice and train the next generation of patient-centered outcomes researchers.	Equitable whole-person care across the lifespan.	Improve health outcomes by promoting high-value, safe, evidence-based, integrated, coordinated, team-based, patient-centered care, with a focus on underserved populations.

High-Level Priorities and Desired Outcomes

A. Health Equity	B. Prevention and Improved Care of Patients With Chronic Conditions	C. Patient, Family, and Provider Experience of Care That Enhances Trust in the Healthcare System	D. High-Quality, Safe Care That Is Aligned With National Health Priorities	E. Primary Care Transformation
Desired Outcomes 1. Reduced health disparities for AHRQ's priority populations 2. Engagement of underrepresented communities in training & implementation initiatives 3. Improved equity in access to needed care	*Desired Outcomes* 1. Increased uptake of evidence-based preventive services, early intervention, and secondary prevention 2. Decreased fragmentation of care for patients with multiple chronic conditions (MCC) 3. Co-design of innovations in care with patients and communities	*Desired Outcomes* 1. Improved patient/family engagement and reported experience of care 2. Focus on whole-person care, with attention to mental health & social determinants of health (SDOH) 3. Improved provider wellness and retention	*Desired Outcomes* 1. Transformation of healthcare organizations into learning health systems 2. Increased uptake of evidence-based practices that strengthen healthcare quality, safety, and value 3. Improved outcomes for targeted national priority conditions	*Desired Outcomes* 1. Uptake of new models of primary care, leveraging digital healthcare 2. Integrated team-based behavioral health 3. Identification and provision of needed resources for comprehensive primary care and uptake of evidence

Cross-cutting Strategies for Achieving Desired Outcomes

- Train and support the next generation of health service researchers with a focus on team science and advancing health equity.
- Develop and maintain the AHRQ infrastructure needed to synthesize and accelerate evidence to practice.
- Leverage and support innovation in digital health, clinical decision support, and new models of care.
- Build data, measurement, and analytic capacity to benchmark and evaluate uptake and use of evidence in learning health systems to improve outcomes that matter to patients.
- Accelerate the uptake of evidence in practice to optimize individual and population health and achieve health equity for all.
- Disseminate evidence to Federal/State/local healthcare decision makers with targeted communication strategies.
- Provide the evidence to inform policy changes needed for sustainable implementation and incorporation of evidence by healthcare systems, practices, and providers.
- Evaluate the impact of PCORTF investments on care delivery, quality, costs, health outcomes, and health disparities.

SOURCE: https://www.ahrq.gov/pcor/strategic-framework/index.html (accessed September 21, 2022).